Aimee K. Cassiday-Shaw, MA

Family Abuse and the Bible

The Scriptural Perspective

*Pre-publication
REVIEWS,
COMMENTARIES,
EVALUATIONS . . .*

"God does have something to say about abuse in the family and Aimee K. Cassiday-Shaw has taken the time to find out what it is. She has given us one of the most important books on the subject that I have read to date. This should be required reading for every member of the church in a time when the family is under the greatest spiritual attack in history. Certainly no biblical counselor should be without this important work."

Pastor Daniel S. Adams, AA, BS
Executive Director/Founder,
Jerusalem House Ministries,
Bethlehem, PA

"Can a Christian husband get away with beating his wife and children, using the Bible to 'justify' his sinful actions? Sadly, a lot of times, yes. This sin-laced blow to the Christian family of the twenty-first century is a steadily growing plague. Aimee K. Cassiday-Shaw sheds light upon how Satan is actively waging war against the Christian family, and choosing abuse as one of his most effective weapons.

Spiritual armor is a necessity for the Christian woman to do her part in the army of God; to fight in this battle Satan has waged. Cassiday-Shaw, through her book *Family Abuse and the Bible*, supplies her readers with the biblical Scripture, statistics, and information necessary to emerge from this battle victorious in the Lord.

Read it and weep, get down on your knees, and then put on the armor of God . . . and fight for what's right."

Mary C. Ross-Geertsema
Journalist, Mahwah, NJ

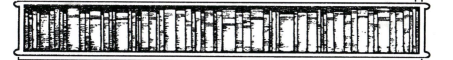

More pre-publication
REVIEWS, COMMENTARIES, EVALUATIONS . . .

"**C**assiday-Shaw has masterfully woven the horrific realities of abuse and the sought-for freedom found in biblical truths to give the reader a rope of hope."

Kathleen Palker
Author of *Spiritual Survival Handbook;*
Creator of Spiritual Survival
for Abuse Survivors
(www.SpiritualSurvival.org)

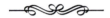

"**C**assiday-Shaw provides the reader with a very realistic perspective on the problems faced within the climate of family abuse. Her insights and solutions are strong and to the point, governed by powerful scriptural insights. A book to be recommended for victims of abuse, those who struggle as abusers, and secondary victims, as well as Christian counselors. A hidden subject opened up very well in the Light."

Mark Stewart, EdD
Instructor, Delta College;
International Student Advisor,
University of the Pacific,
Stockton, CA

"**F**amily Abuse and the Bible is a Christian interpretive commentary on the subjects of family abuse, divorce, marital unity, marital healing, and the American way of being married. It discloses the underlying reasons for the high divorce rate, from a Christian perspective.

Cassiday-Shaw urges those in marriages that are tortured by family abuse to come out of denial. She urges pastors and counselors to help them do so.

This book gives a sound Christian teaching on anger, pointing out that God is slow to anger, and so should we be, as imitators and children of God. Cassiday-Shaw tells us what marriage should be, and also reports what it has tragically become for many who are either victims or perpetrators of domestic violence. She encourages all who have been called to marriage to perceive it in light of God's true Word, and thus take it as seriously as God does."

Ron J. Houssaye, MA
Clinical Social Worker,
Aspira Foster and Family Services,
California Association of Marriage
and Family Therapists

The Haworth Pastoral Press®
An Imprint of The Haworth Press, Inc.
New York • London • Oxford

NOTES FOR PROFESSIONAL LIBRARIANS
AND LIBRARY USERS

This is an original book title published by The Haworth Pastoral Press®, an imprint of The Haworth Press, Inc. Unless otherwise noted in specific chapters with attribution, materials in this book have not been previously published elsewhere in any format or language.

CONSERVATION AND PRESERVATION NOTES

All books published by The Haworth Press, Inc. and its imprints are printed on certified pH neutral, acid free book grade paper. This paper meets the minimum requirements of American National Standard for Information Sciences-Permanence of Paper for Printed Material, ANSI Z39.48-1984.

Family Abuse and the Bible
The Scriptural Perspective

THE HAWORTH PASTORAL PRESS
Religion and Mental Health
Harold G. Koenig, MD
Senior Editor

New, Recent, and Forthcoming Titles:

Adventures in Senior Living: Learning How to Make Retirement Meaningful and Enjoyable by J. Lawrence Driskill

Dying, Grieving, Faith, and Family: A Pastoral Care Approach by George W. Bowman

The Pastoral Care of Depression: A Guidebook by Binford W. Gilbert

Understanding Clergy Misconduct in Religious Systems: Scapegoating, Family Secrets, and the Abuse of Power by Candace R. Benyei

What the Dying Teach Us: Lessons on Living by Samuel Lee Oliver

The Pastor's Family: The Challenges of Family Life and Pastoral Responsibilities by Daniel L. Langford

Somebody's Knocking at Your Door: AIDS and the African-American Church by Ronald Jeffrey Weatherford and Carole Boston Weatherford

Grief Education for Caregivers of the Elderly by Junietta Baker McCall

The Obsessive-Compulsive Disorder: Pastoral Care for the Road to Change by Robert M. Collie

The Pastoral Care of Children by David H. Grossoehme

Ways of the Desert: Becoming Holy Through Difficult Times by William F. Kraft

Caring for a Loved One with Alzheimer's Disease: A Christian Perspective by Elizabeth T. Hall

"Martha, Martha": How Christians Worry by Elaine Leong Eng

Spiritual Care for Children Living in Specialized Settings: Breathing Underwater by Michael F. Friesen

Broken Bodies, Healing Hearts: Reflections of a Hospital Chaplain by Gretchen W. TenBrook

Shared Grace: Therapists and Clergy Working Together by Marion Bilich, Susan Bonfiglio, and Steven Carlson

The Pastor's Guide to Psychiatric Disorders and Mental Health Resources by W. Brad Johnson and William L. Johnson

Christ-Centered Therapy: Empowering the Self by Russ Harris

Bioethics from a Faith Perspective: Ethics in Health Care for the Twenty-First Century by Jack Hanford

Pastoral Counseling: A Gestalt Approach by Ward A. Knights

Family Abuse and the Bible: The Scriptural Perspective by Aimee K. Cassiday-Shaw

When the Caregiver Becomes the Patient: A Journey from a Mental Disorder to Recovery and Compassionate Insight by Daniel L. Langford and Emil J. Authelet

A Theology of God-Talk: The Language of the Heart by J. Timothy Allen

A Practical Guide to Hospital Ministry: Healing Ways by Junietta B. McCall

Pastoral Care for Post-Traumatic Stress Disorder: Healing the Shattered Soul by Dalene Fuller Rogers

Integrating Spirit and Psyche: Using Women's Narratives in Psychotherapy by Mary Pat Henehan

Chronic Pain: Biomedical and Spiritual Approaches by Harold G. Koenig

Family Abuse
and the Bible
The Scriptural Perspective

Aimee K. Cassiday-Shaw, MA

The Haworth Pastoral Press®
An Imprint of The Haworth Press, Inc.
New York • London • Oxford

Published by

The Haworth Pastoral Press®, an imprint of The Haworth Press, Inc., 10 Alice Street, Binghamton, NY 13904-1580.

Disclaimer: Identities and circumstances have been changed to protect confidentiality. There may be sexual or otherwise offensive content, and discretion is advised.

Cover design by Marylouise E. Doyle.

Library of Congress Cataloging-in-Publication Data

Cassiday-Shaw, Aimee K.
 Family abuse and the Bible : the scriptural perspective / Aimee K. Cassiday-Shaw.
  p. cm.
 Includes bibliographical references and index.
 ISBN 0-7890-1576-5 (alk. paper)—ISBN 0-7890-1577-3 (soft : alk. paper)
 1. Family—Biblical teaching. 2. Family—Religious aspects—Christianity. 3. Family violence—Religious aspects—I. Title.

BS680.F3 C37 2002
261.8'327—dc21   2001039710

And this is my prayer: that your love may
abound more and more in knowledge and depth of insight,
so that you may be able to discern what is best
and may be pure and blameless until the day of Christ,
filled with the fruit of righteousness that comes
through Jesus Christ—to the glory and praise of God.

Philippians 1:9-11

ABOUT THE AUTHOR

Aimee K. Cassiday-Shaw, MA, is the founder of Family Abuse Ministries, a not-for-profit organization devoted to bringing a Christian presence into the battered women's movement. Within the ministry, she has developed Bible studies, Bible-based educational models for family abuse, and tracts to be used by law enforcement officers and battered women's shelters. She survived nine years in an abusive marriage. Having earned a bachelor's degree in psychology and a master's degree in criminology, she serves as a social worker in a private foster-family agency. She has spent years counseling batterers in court-ordered treatment programs as well as victims of domestic violence at shelters. She has remarried and has three children. Ms. Cassiday-Shaw is currently pursuing her PhD in conflict management at Trinity Theological Seminary.

CONTENTS

Foreword

Aimee Cassiday-Shaw has raised a new voice to speak out against the pervasive evil of abuse in Christian homes. Voices of protest are desperately needed in light of the many congregations and Christians who minimize, deny, conceal, silence, or ignore the plight of victim, abuser, and innocent children. God has called us to rescue the oppressed from the hand of the violent, but it is much easier to walk by on the other side of the road.

This book is prophetic in its mission of providing evidence, insights, and possible solutions to a problem that few care to address. Unquestionably, Aimee Cassiday-Shaw is a courageous Christian who dares to stand for justice.

I must forthrightly confess that I am not in accord with some of the theological concepts propounded in this book, but in no way does this detract from its value. Precisely because the viewpoint represented is different from that of many others, the work will gain a hearing in a circle that cannot otherwise be penetrated. *Family Abuse and the Bible: The Scriptural Perspective* adds significantly to the body of Christian literature on family abuse precisely because it comes from a very traditional stance often espoused by those who refuse to recognize an ugly and unwelcome reality.

Family abuse happens in all churches, all races, all socioeconomic groups, all neighborhoods, and in all nations. It is there in our midst even when we try to deny it. The real question is: How will people who are obedient to the Word of God deal with oppression, abuse, violence, insult, and injury that is present in every faith community? Our response constitutes a sort of litmus test to a challenge that faces churches everywhere. The Scriptures call for zero tolerance and constructive action, both protective and disciplinary. That call is echoed by this book. May God use it to deliver many from the horrors of domestic abuse.

Catherine Clark Kroeger, PhD
Adjunct Associate Professor
of Classical and Ministry Studies
Gordon-Conwell Theological Seminary
South Hamilton, Massachusetts

Preface

After much thought I decided to write this book. It is not solely based on my experience, although that has certainly played a part in the knowledge I have gained. More important, I believe the writing of this book was directly inspired by God and, therefore, the goal of writing this book is to parallel and amplify God's own words. That is not suggesting that God's words need amplification, because certainly they do not! More simply, our understanding of God's word sometimes is limited, and through amplification, our understanding may be broadened.

This is particularly important regarding the issue of family abuse, a topic largely ignored by the American churches of today. Indeed, sometimes interpretation of Scripture and specific church doctrines can lead to the continuation and justification for family abuse. It is the focus and goal of this book to provide a practical and in-depth study of God's word, and His divine will as it relates to family violence. In addition, this book is written especially for people who have found themselves in abusive relationships. I believe this book will also be beneficial for individuals who work directly with people who have emotional and spiritual issues related to family abuse, as well as to church leaders who may encounter members from their own churches who are living in a hostile environment.

If you are currently living in an abusive environment, or are still in the healing process after having escaped an abusive environment, my hope is that God will reaffirm your experience, reveal His will to you, and speak directly to you through this book. I believe God can and will change your life, and there are three essential steps you can take. First, *open your Bible.* Second, *read this book.* As an even greater benefit, also look up any and all Scriptures contained within it. For clarification and contextual understanding, read several verses prior to and following any Scriptures outlined here. Third, *pray*. Ask Him for guidance, understanding, wisdom, discernment, and protection. Remember to seek Him with a pure heart, and be prepared to follow Him wherever He leads. Understand that sometimes healing cannot occur until the cause of the wound is removed. How, when, and where God does that is unique to your life, but keep in mind as you read this book that how God heals you may not be the way you envisioned it to be. God is, however, the Master Physician—He raised Lazarus from the dead. I think you can trust Him to heal you!

If you are reading this book because you know, have known, or think you will know someone who has experienced family abuse, my hope is that God will speak to you about how to minister to these people. It is always easy to contemplate what choices we think others should make in their lives, but it is sometimes much more difficult to actually walk in their shoes. I hope that reading this book will allow you to understand the depth of emotional and spiritual scarring that occurs within a family that has experienced domestic abuse. I especially hope that this book shows how church doctrine and scriptural understanding can be and have been twisted to allow for the continuation of violence in American homes, and provides a solid biblical basis for offering hope from the freedom of abuse in the Christian marriage.

This book was written employing the use of hermeneutics and contains exegesis of the Scriptures relevant to family abuse. However, this study was not meant to be exhaustive or academic, but biblically sound and easy to read by both lay and scholarly communities. In addition, because research shows a higher rate of female victimization and male perpetration of domestic violence, the subject matter of this book implies gender-based biases. Although family abuse occurs in all contexts possible, for the purposes of this book, a male perpetrator and female victim are assumed in both the language and focus.

Unless otherwise noted, all Scripture is taken from the *New International Version* of the Bible. All references to the Greek and Hebrew original translations are from *Strong's Concordance with Hebrew and Greek-Lexicon*.

SECTION I:
GOD'S DESIGN
FOR FAMILY RELATIONSHIPS

Chapter 1

The Roles of Marriage: Headship and Submission

Perhaps one of the most misunderstood, misinterpreted, and misapplied spiritual principles for marriage is found in Ephesians 5:22 and Colossians 3:18. The apostle Paul wrote in Ephesians 5:22:

Wives, submit to your husbands as to the Lord.

Likewise, in Colossians 3:18 he wrote:

Wives, submit to your husbands, as is fitting in the Lord.

Paul reiterates this principle for us twice, once to the Church at Ephesus, and then again to the Church at Colosse, so this is an important aspect of the husband-wife relationship from God's point of view. Let us look closer at the first Scripture.

"Wives," Paul says. He is writing this specifically to wives. Thus, women and wives must pay close attention to Paul's instruction here. Once Paul has their attention, he continues, "submit to your husbands *as to the Lord.*" The last part of this verse is highlighted because it is the qualifier here. Paul gives wives two instructions: they should submit to their husbands, *and,* they should to the Lord. In fact, Paul assumes the wife is already in submission to the Lord. The phrase "as to" implies that the wife's relationship with the Lord is the example of how she should be in submission to her husband. This portion of the verse tells wives that the nature of their personal relationship with the Lord is the example of the wife's role in the husband-wife relationship. Let's take a closer look at what submission means.

The *Random House Dictionary* defines "submit," first, as a verb. Thus, it is an action. It is something that we do. The first definition given is "to yield (oneself) to the power or authority of another" (p. 1895). Power and yielding are the key concepts in this definition. Another definition given for "submit" is "to present for the approval, consideration, or decision of another" (p. 1895). Ultimately submission means that we yield to the ultimate authority of the person we are in submission to, but also that we present our opinions and ideas to that person for consideration. Our voice is important—so important, in fact, that submission cannot occur unless our opinions are expressed. This point speaks more to the husband's role in the relationship, whether he considers his wife's opinions and ideas, and how he responds to them.

Strong's Greek Concordance defines "submit," or *hupotasso,* as it is translated in both referenced verses as "to arrange under," "to subordinate," and further clarifies it as "a Greek military term meaning 'to arrange [troop divisions] in a military fashion under the command of a leader.' In non-military use, it was "a voluntary attitude of giving in, cooperating, assuming responsibility, and carrying a burden." This is different from the usage of the word "slave" or *doulos,* which is also translated as "servant."

The first part of God's inspired instruction to wives is to submit to their husbands (not be slaves to), and He uses the wife's personal relationship with Jesus as the model of how this should be done. He continues in Ephesians 5:23 to write:

For the husband is the head of the wife, as Christ is the head of the church, his body, of which he is the Savior.

Again, let us take an in-depth look at what God is saying to both husbands and wives here. "For the husband is the head of the wife." In other words, the husband is in charge, the head, the leader in the marriage. This point causes a lot of division and strife not only among husbands and wives, but also among believers and nonbelievers. With the modern influence of feminism and women's rights, many women have become offended at this spiritual principle, which has, in turn, caused them to be repulsed by Christianity. The word "obey," which is a synonym for "submit," was a traditional vow made from a wife to her husband in the wedding ceremony. That word has been replaced as the concepts behind it have been grossly distorted and misinterpreted in modern society.

Some women may think their lives would be easier if God does not literally mean what He says in the foregoing Scripture. When misunderstood in context, it is a difficult principle to adhere to. However, the husband is the head of the wife—or at least should be. If we go on to read the rest of that sentence, "as Christ is head of the church," God gives the example of how a husband is the head of the wife. This time, however, He is not using her personal relationship with Jesus as an example of her role in marriage. He is almost stepping back and saying, "Look at the relationship of Jesus to the church. That is the example of how your husband is the head of you." In other words, the relationship of the church to Jesus should have the same characteristics as the wife's relationship to her husband. To examine this further, we have to closely look at the example God is providing. What is the church's relationship to Jesus? God gives us a little clue when He states that the church is Jesus' "body, of which he is the Savior." This directly tells us that the church is His body, which is supported by other Scriptures (Romans 12:5, 1 Corinthians 12:12+, Ephesians 1:22-23, Ephesians 5:30, Colossians 1:24). Furthermore, He is the Savior of that body. Thus, wives are like the body of their husbands, and the husband is like the wife's savior. We are treading through deep waters here, so we must approach interpretations carefully, and with full contextual knowledge of God's character. First and foremost, we must keep in mind that Jesus is our Savior. He is the one who paid the price for our salvation, and the one who is due the glory for that. Take a closer look at what it means to be a Savior.

Paul, from prison, writes to the Church at Philippi about the character of Jesus. He instructs them, "Your attitude should be the same as that of Christ Jesus: Who, being in very nature God, did not consider equality with God something to be grasped, but made himself nothing, taking the very nature of a servant, being made in human likeness. And being found in appearance as a man, he humbled himself and became obedient to death—even death on a cross!" (Philippians 2:5-8). The concepts here are servanthood and humility, not power and authority. We read in that passage that God exalted His Son in demonstration of the spiritual principle of obedience. Power and authority are not in opposition to servanthood and humility, but in the spiritual Kingdom, power and authority are the natural consequences of servanthood and humility. "For whoever exalts himself will be humbled, and whoever humbles himself will be exalted" (Matthew 23:12; see also Luke 14:11, Isaiah 26:5).

Now that we have a clearer idea of what it means to be a Savior, let's return to the Ephesians passage. Although Paul starts out clearly speaking to wives, he is using the metaphor of the church's relationship to Jesus as an example of the wife's relationship to her husband. He strengthens this teaching further in Ephesians 5:24:

> Now as the church submits to Christ, so also wives should submit to their husbands in everything.

While He is asking the wives to think of marriage in those terms, He is also giving indirect instruction to the husbands as to their role in the marriage. The wife submits to the husband, but the husband is elevated to the position of head. That is not only an honor; it denotes a huge amount of responsibility on the husband. This will become clearer as we examine the entire Ephesians context. Unfortunately, many people misinterpret Scripture because they fail to see the entire context within which God is speaking. If we look at just one part of the Jesus-church relationship, or of the husband-wife relationship, we fail to understand how one is dependent on the other. In other words, although God is giving a specific instruction to wives, He is also implying that this instruction operates within an outline for marriage that He designed. He tells us in Genesis 2:24 that Adam and Eve, as husband and wife, "will become one flesh." Thus, while each partner in the relationship is an individual, has an individual relationship with God, and is accountable as an individual to God, He designed each to function in perfect harmony as one if they both follow His outline. If either one of the two fails to follow God's marital plan, the marriage is not God-centered, and may be subject to fail. Again, we are treading through deep waters and must be careful. The Ephesians passage further says that the wife should submit to the husband "in everything." Although some people may use this to argue that a wife must submit to her husband regardless of whether her husband is fulfilling God's expectation of his role in the marriage, we need to look closer at God's precise wording here. Notice that He does not say "always," or "in every circumstance." He specifically says "in everything." God is saying that we do not pick and choose what we will submit to. In context, He is saying this with the assumption that the wife and husband are in a "right" relationship. Remember, this is His perfect plan for marriage. He is talking to wives who are in a marriage that is based on the outline He has given. This corresponds with what He writes in Colossians 3:18:

> Wives, submit to your husbands, as is fitting in the Lord.

Here is the qualifier of His instruction: "as is fitting in the Lord." In other words, He is saying that in a "right" relationship the wife's submission is in conjunction, is aligned with, her submission to the Lord. These wives, He is saying, must submit themselves in everything because through that submission to their husbands, they are in submission to Him. For wives who find themselves in a marriage that is not based on God's outline, He is not saying that they must submit to a husband who abuses them. Again, we must be extremely careful whenever we are deciding which situation a particular Scripture may apply to. A deep understanding of the nature of God, the immediate context of what He is saying, and an entire knowledge of His word is required. Keeping that in mind, let us read on in Ephesians.

After Paul gives his instructions to wives, he gives a very specific instruction to husbands. He writes in Ephesians 5:25:

> Husbands, love your wives, just as Christ loved the church and gave himself up for her—

Now Paul is asking for the attention of husbands and, just like he did with the wives, he is giving a very specific instruction. Again, God uses the church-Jesus relationship as a metaphor to teach a fundamental principle of His design for marriage. This time, however, He is focusing on the husband's role in that relationship. Remember, the wife represents the church, and her role, just as the church's role, is in submission to her husband, who represents Jesus. Now, we turn to the husbands, and God asks them to "love your wives." This love that God is asking of husbands is not a human love; it is not a romantic love; it is not a friendship love. It is *the* love of God Himself. The original Greek word that appears in this portion of the biblical text is *agapao,* or agape love. Again, agape love is expressed through His word as *the love of God.* It is distinguished from four other types of love expressed throughout God's word. These four other types of love are human expressions of love, but agape love is a reflection of God's love for us. It is the purest form of love. This agape love is illustrated, again through a metaphor, when Paul writes in Ephesians 5:25: "just as Christ loved the church and gave himself up for her." In other words, God is saying to husbands, "I want you to love your wife just like Jesus loves His church, and you demonstrate that love by giving yourself up for her, just like Jesus gave Himself up for His church."

Headship in this context no longer seems to be a position of authority or power as it may have when we thought of headship in the context of submission. Indeed, God's definition of the husband's role implies a mutual submission in the marital relationship. The husband is supposed to love his wife by "giving himself up for her." That certainly seems to denote a sacrifice on the husband's part. While sacrifice and submission are not the same, one cannot make a sacrifice without being in submission to something. Indeed, sacrifice and submission seem to be two sides of the same coin. It is also interesting to note, as we look at the entirety of the context within which Paul was writing, that in the verse prior to instructing wives to submit to their husbands, he wrote:

Submit to one another out of reverence for Christ (Ephesians 5:21, italics added).

It seems more than mere coincidence that of all the places in the letter that Paul could have placed that instruction, he placed it immediately before he instructed wives to submit to their husbands. It also seems more than mere coincidence that Paul's instruction to wives is very similar in both Ephesians and Colossians, but when we compare his instruction to husbands, Paul adds an element. Let us examine the Colossians 3:19 passage:

Husbands, love your wives and do not be harsh with them.

"Do not be harsh with them." That seems to be much more direct than the Ephesians verse. Perhaps the church at Colosse was having problems with husbands abusing their "authority" of the marital relationship and were being harsh with their wives. Assuming for a moment that that is the case, let us take a look again at the preceding Colossians verse:

Wives, submit to your husbands, as is fitting in the Lord (Colossians 3:18).

Again, notice the qualifier He gives: *as is fitting in the Lord.* Why would Paul write here, "in the Lord," when he wrote to the Ephesian women "to the Lord." It seems that Paul is giving two different directions, although they are within the same spiritual principle. Although this distinction may seem irrelevant, in light of the context, it is very relevant. The root Greek word that was translated as "fitting" in this verse is *aneko,* and it is also translated as "convenient" in Ephesians 5:4 and Philemon 1:8. That is especially interesting when you consider that these are the only three occurrences of this word in the entire Bible! So, Paul seems to be telling these Christian women whose husbands may have treated them harshly that they must submit to their husbands *but* only if it is convenient. Now, before we get carried away with this idea, let us examine what exactly He may mean by convenient, or fitting. First, He does not say "as is fitting to you." He says "as is fitting *in the Lord.*" Second, He does not say "to the Lord." He says very specifically "*in* the Lord." So, we can gather that God is saying to these wives who may have had harsh husbands, "I want you to submit to your husbands, but if your husband is not in submission to Me, and your marital relationship is not operating *in* Me, then your submission to your husband may not be fitting with what I am asking of you." To illustrate this, reflect back to the earlier discussion on the definition of submission. Remember that submission requires one "to present as an opinion." Stop and think about that for a minute. Why would submission require you to present your opinion to the person you are in submission to? Well, before we can determine if we are in agreement or opposition, we have to present our opinion on the matter. If we are in agreement, we really do not need to submit. In fact, it is only when we find ourselves in a disagreement that submission becomes a possibility.

To put this in a spiritual perspective, God is saying that when a husband is in submission to Him, that husband is the head of his family, and the wife should submit to her husband because it is convenient for her to do so. Now, not all wives would agree with that. In fact, many Christian wives struggle with the very idea of submission or, at least, with their ability to do it gracefully. Although God said "in everything" a wife must submit, He may have specified this to Christian wives who find it difficult to submit to their husbands in day-to-day decision making. There is a big difference between the wife who is uncomfortable being called to submit to her husband when he feels led by the Lord to take on a new job, and the wife who finds herself in the predicament of whether she should submit to her husband who clearly is not following the Lord. More will be said about applying the principle of submission in our relationships; for now we just need to acknowledge that God's word is a living word and, thus, speaks to us as within our individual situations. One person's ability to apply a certain spiritual principle in his or her life at any given moment does not serve as a rule that another person must apply that same principle . A mature Christian walk requires a knowledge of God's entire word, as well as the wisdom to apply it to our lives. With that in mind, let us turn to a discussion on man's and woman's place in God's awesome design for us.

Chapter 2

The Nature of Woman:
Woman As the Vulnerable Partner

We know that God asks wives to submit to their husbands, but what about the role of women in general? Paul elaborates again on the role of women when he writes to the Church at Corinth. This time he is not writing just to wives, but to a general audience that included the entire church. Paul writes to the Corinthians, as recorded in 1 Corinthians 11:3:

> Now I want you to realize that the head of every man is Christ, and the head of the woman is man, and the head of Christ is God.

Again, we see the central theme of God's design. There is a hierarchy, with God at the top. Knowing that He is a merciful, wise, loving, and forgiving God, we may not mind God being at the top, but women may be left asking: "Why, God, did you put him as the head of me?" This may be especially true for women who have found themselves in relationships with men, whether they be fathers, husbands, boyfriends, brothers, or even sons, who have been less than edifying. It is not the goal of this book to focus on a debate as to whether women or men are superior, but to point out what God says about the subject. Women need to understand, and accept that God has established an order, and there are clear reasons why. Men also need to understand that they are placed at the top of that order in terms of human relationships, but that they are not at *the* top. They must be accountable to God. In order to understand the full scheme, we need to start from the beginning. In the book of Genesis, we read the story of creation.

The first verse that appears in the Bible that reveals to us our place within God's creation of the world is found in Genesis 1:26. God says:

> Let us make man in our image, in our likeness, and let *them* rule over the fish of the sea and the birds of the air, over the livestock, over all the earth, and over all the creatures that move along the ground [italics added].

"Them," as it appears in the above Scripture, refers to many men. God knew man would multiply, so He was referring to the many men who would inhabit the earth. God's first distinction between man and woman comes in the very next verse but, interestingly, it comes before He even describes the process of how He created man and woman. He says in Genesis 1:27:

> So God created man in his own image, in the image of God he created *him;* male and female he created *them* [italics added].

Keep in mind that this distinction God made between man and woman does not mean that man and woman are separate in God's eyes. In terms of gender, God makes no distinction between man and woman. We know this from Paul's letter to the church at Corinth: "In the Lord, however, woman is not independent of man, nor is man independent of woman. For as woman came from man, so also man is born of woman. But everything comes from God" (1 Corinthians 11:11-12). We will read later in Genesis that Adam and Eve became "one."

We could spend an entire book talking about the intricacies of God's plan as revealed in the creation story. Please read Genesis to gain a full knowledge of God's creation story. The key points that should be noted are that God indeed formed man, Adam, first, and that after some period of time it became apparent that Adam needed a helper. Then God created woman, Eve. Not only did woman come after man, she came from man. Literally. Her sole purpose for creation seems for her to be a "helper" (Genesis 2:20b).

So, not only was man created first, woman was created as a helper for man, and she was created from him. Thus, as Paul writes in 1 Corinthians 11:7-9:

—since he [man] is the image and glory of God; but the woman is the glory of man. For man did not come from woman, but woman from man; neither was man created for woman, but woman for man.

Again, we see a clear order established by God. Now, we need to focus on why this order may have been established. The central reason is outlined by the apostle Peter, when he wrote in 1 Peter 3:7b:

—treat them [wives] with respect as the *weaker* partner and as heirs with you of the gracious gift of life—[italics added].

We will revisit this verse later, but for now the focus is on Peter's claim that women are weaker than men. Let us keep in mind he is writing within a context of the "partnership" of the husband and wife relationship. Was Peter sexist in assuming that the wife is weaker because she is a woman? Peter's use of the word "weaker," or the Greek word *asthenes,* literally translates as "weak, infirm, and feeble." According to *Strong's Concordance,* it is commonly translated as "sick." Although women are generally physically weaker than men because of physiological design, the predominant use of the word implies a spiritual weakness (see Matthew 26:41; Romans 5:6; 1 Corinthians 4:10). To illustrate this, let us turn again to the creation account in Genesis.

God had instructed Adam not to eat a certain fruit from a certain tree within the Garden of Eden (Genesis 2:16-17). The account does not specifically tell us that God instructed Eve not to eat the fruit. In Genesis 2:16 it says "God commanded *the man."* Indeed, it is not until verse 18 that the idea that God should create a woman for the man is even mentioned. We must assume that Eve at some point knew about God's command, because in Genesis 3, the serpent asked Eve if God had really commanded that they not eat the fruit and she replied that He did. In Genesis 3:6 we read that Eve "took some and ate it. She also gave some to her husband, who was with her, and he ate it." So, they *both* disobeyed God. They both ate the fruit that God had forbidden them to eat. How did that happen? In the beginning of Genesis 3, we read that a serpent (Satan) appeared to Eve and lied to her. He basically told Eve that what God had told her was untrue, and presented the fruit to her in such a way as to lead her to believe it would be a benefit for her to eat it. Eve was deceived. Her fatal mistake was that she believed the lie of the enemy. This is where the spiritual weakness of woman first manifested itself.

Chapter 3

The Nature of Man:
Man As the Responsible Partner

If woman is clearly the more vulnerable gender, we would assume that man is the stronger gender. If we assume that man is the stronger gender, we also have to assume that man is more accountable. More is expected of man because more has been given to him ("and from the one who has been entrusted with much, much more will be asked," Luke 12:48b). If a man and a woman are running a race, and the woman, because of her nature is slower, then we would expect the man to win that race. So the man's strength places him as head of the woman, but also gives him more responsibility. Remember, like Eve, Adam also ate of the fruit that God told them not to. While Eve ate the forbidden fruit first, God recounts that she was deceived by the enemy. He also reiterates this through Paul in 1 Timothy 2:14, where Paul writes:

> And Adam was not the one deceived; it was the woman who was deceived and became a sinner.

Yes, Eve was deceived. God alludes that the serpent was a very beautiful creature. The serpent certainly did not present himself in a way that would cause one to automatically distrust him. In fact, Paul tells us in 2 Corinthians 11:14 that "Satan himself masquerades as an angel of light." It is no wonder Eve was deceived. The Genesis account also tells us that the serpent "was more crafty than any of the wild animals the Lord God had made" (Genesis 3:1). Eve was up against a very treacherous being. It is probably more than mere coincidence that Satan presented himself to her first, and not to Adam. He must have already known that she was the more vulnerable partner. What about Adam? It almost seems that Adam is getting off the hook when Paul writes that "the woman—became a sinner" (1 Timothy 2:14). Adam did eat of the fruit too.

We read further in Genesis 3 that after Adam and Eve ate the fruit, God was in the garden and He spoke to Adam. He asked Adam, not Eve, "Have you eaten from the tree that I commanded you not to eat from?" (Genesis 3:11b). Adam's response, while tragic in context, is almost humorous. Adam does not answer with a simple "yes" or "no." He answers with an excuse. He answers with a justification, a rationalization, and he even displaces the blame for his own actions. He said to God, "The woman you put here with me—" (Genesis 3:12). To paraphrase Adam's response to God, Adam was saying, "If it hadn't been for that woman you gave me, Lord. It's all her fault. You should've never given me that woman." That is hardly the way Adam felt about Eve at first. Remember Adam's reaction when he saw Eve for the first time? He said, "This is now bone of my bone and flesh of my flesh—" (Genesis 2:23). Adam apparently felt very connected and bonded with Eve. But, as soon as things go wrong, Adam instantly separates himself from Eve. He no longer wants to take the responsibility that she is "bone of his bones and flesh of his flesh." Not only does Adam forget that Eve and he are "one flesh" (Genesis 2:24), he does not want to be accountable to God. God directly commanded Adam, not Eve, not to eat the fruit of the tree. God created Adam as the head of his wife. Along with his creation came a certain degree of responsibility over her. We read that Adam was there with Eve when she ate the fruit. Why did he not speak up? After they had eaten the fruit, God came into the garden and spoke directly to Adam, not Eve. In fact, God came and specifically called for Adam. Where was Adam? In Genesis 3:8 we read that Adam and Eve "hid from the Lord God among the trees in the garden." While they both ate and both hid, Eve was under the leadership of her husband. Here lies the first manifestation of the lack of accountability of man.

We clearly see the nature of Adam and Eve and the implications their actions had for us as a race, as well as for each gender. Thank God for the entirety of His plan, in that He sent his Son to redeem us from our sinful nature. Paul wrote, "For just as through the disobedience of the one man [Adam] the many were made sinners, so also through the obedience of the one man [Jesus] the many will be made righteous" (Romans 5:19). However, we must live with the reality that Jesus came to justify us, and not to eradicate sin. Our Christian faith is that He will return and when He does He will set things right. In the meantime, we are living within the framework of our sinful human nature, as first manifested through the account of Adam and Eve at the Garden of Eden.

Hopefully through that account, and other Scriptures God has given us, we better understand His perfect design for marriage and partnership, the man's and woman's roles in that relationship, and also the inherent problems we encounter within those roles. Just as Jesus is our model of God's perfect design of a sinless human existence, so also are Adam and Eve (prior to their sin) a model of God's perfect design for marriage. However, just as we recognize that because of our sinful nature we can never attain perfection as Jesus demonstrated it on this earth, we must also recognize that we cannot have marriages that represent the perfection of Adam and Eve's marriage before they sinned. That is not to say we should not try. Indeed, we call upon God daily to guide us on the path toward His perfect will. At the same time, we have to be aware that God's plan for marriage is a dynamic and interdependent plan, and that a breakdown in any one aspect of the plan, process, or role of the players will lead to destruction. We live in the reality of our powerlessness. We cannot force another person to be accountable to God any more than Eve had control over Adam, or Adam had control over Eve. Through this understanding we have to accept that woman and man, even though they may be united in marriage, are spiritually separated from each other because of the original sin. This was not God's perfect plan for the way marriage should be.

However, we have a hope. That hope, not only as an individual, but also as a husband and wife, is Jesus Christ. Indeed, the only way for a man and woman to be spiritually united is through Jesus Christ. Jesus, praying to His Father, said: "—that they may be one as we are one: I in them and you in me. May they be brought to complete unity—" (John 17:22-23). Although Jesus was praying for all believers, He certainly alludes to a fundamental spiritual principle: we all, as believers, whether husband and wife, or brother and sister, need to be united in Him. That requires a spiritual fellowship with Him first. We cannot have unity without having something in common to unite us. That is where the marital breakdown can and does occur. God not only recognized this, He spent a great deal of time speaking about it, as we will examine later. Before we go any further into the marital relationship, let us take a brief look at the parental role God prescribed to parents.

Chapter 4

God's Design for Parenthood: Spare Not the Rod

It has been a Christian tradition not only to quote, but adhere to the following popular verse:

> He who spares the rod hates his son, but he who loves him is careful to discipline him (Proverbs 13:24).

This verse is often paraphrased: "Spare the rod, spoil the child." It is tragic that this and other verses have been taken literally to mean that parents should beat their children in the name of discipline. Is that what God meant? There is hardly any question about God's stand on discipline. Indeed, if parents consistently withhold discipline, God basically tells us that their children will "die." When we read the word "rod" as it consistently appears in reference to discipline, we tend to assume that God is implying a literal rod that we beat children with. A thorough study on the original language of biblical text tells us what God may have meant. "Rod" appears in the Bible many times. The original Hebrew word that has often been translated as "rod" is *shebet*. That same word has also been translated as "staff," "correction," "discipline," and most interestingly, as "tribe." This same word, shebet, appears in many other verses. Let us take a look at a few of them as they relate to discipline:

> Folly is bound up in the heart of a child, but the rod of discipline will drive it far from him (Proverbs 22:15).

Do not withhold discipline from a child; if you punish him with the rod, he will not die (Proverbs 23:13).

The rod of correction imparts wisdom, but a child left to himself disgraces his mother (Proverbs 29:15).

Discipline your son, for in that there is hope; do not be a willing party to his death (Proverbs 19:18).

These verses tell us about God's design for parents and children. Perhaps the harshest of these verses is Proverbs 23:13. The King James translation replaces the word "punish" with the word "beatest," so that the King James Version (KJV) reads: "Withhold not correction from the child; for if thou beatest him with the rod, he shall not die." Did God literally mean that we should beat children to prevent them from death? To answer this question we must first examine what God may have meant when He said "he [a child] will not die" if we punish him.

Death, as most often referred to in the Scriptures, does not imply mere physical death, but death in the sense of eternal spiritual separation from God after we die in our physical bodies. In other words, death is often implied in Scriptures as a state of being in hell. We, as Christians, although we die a physical death, have eternal life with God through Jesus (1 John 5:11). Anything other than that is a permanent death, or separation from God. That is hell. Indeed, the KJV of Proverbs 23:14 states, "Thou shalt beat him with the rod, and shalt deliver his soul from hell." Thus, it is not a physical death we are trying to spare our children from, but a spiritual death, an eternal separation from God. Anyone who has children knows that we do not have to teach our children to disobey. It is an inherent aspect of their nature. Stop and think about a child at two years old: rebellious, strong-willed, and disobedient. No one has taught children to be that way; they are born that way. However, we do have to teach them *not* to be that way. How do we do that? We "do not spare the rod." In other words, we save our children from their own demise through discipline. Before we look at the specific instruction to parents, let us explore discipline in a more general context.

Several verses refer to the discipline of God. Indeed, from all scriptural accounts, God is a punishing and disciplining God. Is there a difference between discipline and punishment? In action, perhaps not, but in heart there may be a big difference. Indeed, the Old Testament often paints God as a punishing God. Destruction by God's hand fell upon those who were rebellious. The New Testament, however, paints God through Jesus as a God of loving discipline. We must keep in mind that God is never changing. He is the God of the Old and New Testaments. Something, however, did change. Jesus was sent to die on a cross for our sins. With that, He reiterated the loving discipline of God. Much is written about this discipline. In Revelation 3:19, the Lord Himself spoke to the apostle John in a vision. He told John to write to the church at Laodicea that "those whom I love I rebuke and discipline." If we truly examine the context of what God is saying here, we see that love and discipline are like two sides of the same coin. We are disciplined by our heavenly father because He loves us. As parents, we discipline our own children because we love them. At least, that is how it should be. There is a distinction, however, between love and punishment. John writes in 1 John 4:18:

> There is no fear in love. But perfect love drives out fear, because fear has to do with punishment. The one who fears is not made perfect in love.

Fear is the key here. It is the element that distinguishes discipline from punishment. Before we examine other verses pertaining to the discipline of God, let us look closer at fear. King Solomon wrote in the book of Proverbs:

> The fear of the Lord is the beginning of knowledge, but fools despise wisdom and discipline (Proverbs 1:7).

Notice that both fear and discipline appear in this same verse. That may seem contradictory to what John wrote later (1 John

4:18). The original word for "fear" has a different definition in each of these verses. The "fear" in Solomon's verse is the Hebrew word *yirah,* which has been translated to express "respect," "reverence," and "piety," whereas the "fear" used in John's verse is the Greek word *phobos,* for a literal translation of "fear," "dread," and "terror" *(Strong's Concordance).* Thus, the Proverbs 1:7 verse is not implying a literal fear as it relates to punishment, but rather a respect, reverence, and awe of God. Discipline is never to be feared. This is because we know it comes from love. That does not mean that we like it. In fact, it is written in Hebrews:

> No discipline seems pleasant at the time, but painful. Later on, however, it produces a harvest of righteousness and peace for those who have been trained by it" (Hebrews 12:11).

Discipline is painful. It is not pleasant. However, notice that it produces not only righteousness, but peace. It gives us a sense that we are loved. To understand this from a biblical context, we have to relate it back to God's use of the word "rod" when He shares with us about His will in terms of discipline. In the oft quoted twenty-third Psalm, David writes:

> The Lord is my shepherd—your rod and your staff, they comfort me (Psalms 23:1, 4c).

This entire Psalm paints a picture of a shepherd and his sheep. Indeed, God refers to us, His people, several times as sheep (Numbers 27:17, Psalms 100:3, Jeremiah 50:6, Ezekiel 34:11, John 10:14, John 10:27, plus many more). We, like David, are the sheep and He is the shepherd. When we examine what shepherds do, and what they use their staffs for, we get a more complete understanding of how God relates this to discipline. A shepherd uses his rod to protect his sheep by fighting off wild animals, and he uses his staff to guide straying sheep. Thus, God uses His rod and staff as a metaphor for the spiritual principles of discipline. What is God's "rod"? We can conceive of a rod as being like a sword, and God specifically tells us that His sword is His word (Ephesians 6:17, Hebrews 4:12, Revelation 1:16, Revelation 2:12). Thus, the word of God is not only the "rod" with which we are disciplined, but it is also the "rod" with which we, as parents, discipline our own children. It is a stern but loving rod, meant to keep the sheep from going off the path. This is what God implies in Proverbs 22:6:

> Train a child in the way he should go, and when he is old he will not turn from it.

Indeed, God's discipline, while sovereign and divine, is an example of how our discipline toward our children should be. Just like the Jesus-church relationship represents God's perfect will for the husband-wife relationship, so also the shepherd-sheep relationship represents God's perfect will for the parent-child relationship. Now, does the shepherd beat his sheep? If he did, would they follow him, would they respect him, or have loyalty toward him? Probably not. That is why Paul writes twice about the consequence of the shepherd not taking proper care of his sheep. He instructs us in Ephesians 6:4:

> Fathers, do not exasperate your children; instead, bring them up in the training and instruction of the Lord.

Just as when Paul was directing his instruction to husbands and wives, he is now specifically addressing fathers. That is not suggesting that fathers are the only parents worth addressing. Certainly mothers are just as responsible for discipline as are fathers. However, remember the discussion on the roles of men and women in God's perfect design. In families where a man is present, the man is the head of that family. The man is the shepherd of his family. The shepherd is responsible to guide the sheep. That is not to say that the wife is a sheep in her husband's flock. Remember, scriptures tell us that women are "weaker," but that they are equal partners in God's eyes (1 Peter 3:7, 1 Corinthians 11:11). So, we are all sheep of the Lord's flock, just like our children are sheep of our flock. Shepherding is a mutual responsibility of the mother and the father, but the man is the stronger shepherd, which makes him the "head shepherd." Single-parent families can and do function because the sheep only need one shepherd, but the sheep are much more protected when there are two shepherds looking after them. So, while Paul is addressing fathers, this particular instruction applies to mothers, and anyone else who is in a parental role with children.

In this Ephesians verse Paul tells parents not to exasperate their children. The KJV of this same verse reads: "And, ye fathers, provoke not your children to wrath—." The King James translation gives an indication that to exasperate means not only to provoke, but to provoke to wrath. In a commentary on Colossians 3:21, which will be addressed shortly, Matthew Henry writes: "Let not your authority over them [your children] be exercised with rigor and severity, but with kindness and gentleness, lest you raise their passions and discourage them in their duty, and by holding the reins too tight make them fly out with greater fierceness" (Henry, 2000, p. 2335).

God instructs parents what not to do. In the second part of Ephesians 6:4, He also instructs parents what they should do: "bring them up in the training and instruction of the Lord." The training and instruction of the Lord is given by His word: the rod, the sword, the staff. Again, the rod in "beatest with the rod" (Proverbs 23:13 KJV) is often taken literally to mean a physical rod, but it actually may mean a spiritual rod. This is even more evident when we compare the above NIV translation of Ephesians 6:4 with the KJV, which reads: "—but bring them up in the nurture and admonition of the Lord." We are to raise our children with the nurture and training, instruction and admonition of the Lord. Likewise, Paul wrote to the Church at Colosse, as recorded in Colossians 3:21:

Fathers, do not embitter your children, or they will become discouraged.

Like Paul did with the husbands and wives, he gives a second instruction in two letters to two distinct churches. This time Paul does not just give a "do not/do" instruction, but a "cause/effect" instruction. He writes that if fathers (parents) embitter their children, the children will become discouraged. The original Greek word for "discouraged" *(athumeo)* is further translated as "to be dis-heartened, dispirited, broken in spirit." Thus, it is clear that we should not discourage or enrage our children. Does God give any more instruction to parents about what they should do? The answer is yes. God tells us in Deuteronomy 6:6-7:

> These commandments that I give you today are to be upon your hearts. Impress them on your children. Talk about them when you sit at home and when you walk along the road, when you lie down and when you get up.

What a beautiful Scripture! God says to take His commandments (His "rod") and "impress" them on our children. Impress. Not beat into, but impress. God even tells us how we do that: "talk about them." Spend quality time with our children, sitting at home, walking along the road, maybe stopping along the way to admire the beautiful colors of a nearby flower, and the awe of His creations. There probably is not anything more impressive to children than their parents spending quality time nurturing their spirits.

We all know there are times when children need more than just a mere walk along the road. In keeping with God's balanced character, He tells us to punish, teach, correct, and discipline our children, but He also tells us not to do it with undue harshness, but rather with the wisdom and instruction of the Master Shepherd. Again, when we think in the terms God offers, it is difficult to argue for the spanking of children. That is because it is difficult to imagine the Lord hitting us, and it is impossible to imagine the Lord beating us. The difference between the two is drastic to some, but can be very subtle if based on outward appearance. Whether you should spank your child is ultimately a personal choice. Just keep in mind not the specific punishment, but the state of the parent's heart when discipline is being carried out. In a commentary on Proverbs 23:12-16, Matthew Henry (2000) states, "For the present [discipline] is not joyous, but grievous, both to the parent and the child; but when it is *given with wisdom, designed for good, accompanied with prayer, and blessed of God,* it may prove a happy means of preventing his [the child's] utter destruction and delivering his soul from hell" (p. 1007, italics added).

Chapter 5

The Child's Role:
The Fifth Commandment

We cannot discuss family relationships without some discussion on the child's relationship to the parent(s) in the family. Through understanding God's entire plan for us, we can better comprehend how our own lives, and our own families, function within (or without) His design. This understanding gives us a measuring rod to gauge ourselves and our family relationships. God's most apparent measuring rod for children is found in Exodus 20:12, where He gives His fifth commandment:

> Honor your father and your mother, so that you may live long in the land the Lord your God is giving you.

What does it mean to "honor"? The original Hebrew word that appears in Exodus 20:12, which has been translated as "honor," is *kabad* and it has two definitions: "to make heavy, make dull, make insensible," and "to make honorable, honor, glorify." Because God implies that honor is an action, it must be a verb. The *Random House Webster's Unabridged Dictionary* defines the verb "honor" as "to hold in high respect" (p. 918). That is the command that God lays out specifically for children. They should honor, glorify, and respect their parent(s). But, keeping in mind the discussion in the previous section, respect is earned. Although God is not giving children any qualifier in His instructions here, He implies one through the Scriptures we discussed in the previous section. Remember, God instructed parents to "impress" His commands on their children's hearts (Deuteronomy 6:7). Isn't that how honor and respect are earned, through impressing those who honor and respect us?

This spiritual principle and the dynamics of God's perfect design for families are interdependent. In other words, the child has a role and responsibility to God to fulfill His outline of that role, but that is not independent of the role He lays out for parents. Parents also have a responsibility, and much more accountability. Just as the husband is more accountable because he is the "head," so also are parents more accountable because they are the "head" of the child. Before we assume that God is holding parents completely accountable for their children's actions, let us look at what He says in Deuteronomy 24:16:

> Father shall not be put to death for their children, nor children put to death for their fathers; each is to die for his own sin.

God tells us through the full picture of these Scriptures that parents are responsible for their own actions, and for gently guiding their children ("sheep") on the right path. If the sheep continually rebel and refuse to be gently corrected back onto the path, they are responsible for their own disobedience. However, parents can actually run their sheep off the path when their discipline is of the wrong motive or heart.

Again, we see that although a hierarchy exists there is mutual interdependence. It is like a chain in that each link is necessary to make up the strength of the entire chain. If a link within the chain is not doing what it is supposed to do, the links after it, or before it, are unlikely to do what they are supposed to do and, hence, we have a "chain reaction." Each link depends on the others, but is also an individual that receives personal strength from God. This is how families operate both within God's design and also within our fleshly, sinful nature.

Providing that all the other links in the chain are strong, a child is completely accountable to God to fulfill His commands. In addition to the original Exodus commandment, Paul writes in the New Testament:

Children, obey your parents in the Lord, for this is right (Ephesians 6:1).

Children, obey your parents in everything, for this pleases the Lord (Colossians 3:20).

Notice again, as with the wives, Paul writes in Ephesians "obey your parents in the Lord." This is almost exactly what he wrote to the wives at Colosse. This implies an assumption that the child's parents are operating within a relationship and obedience to the Lord. For children, obedience to their parents is the same as obedience to the Lord. What happens when the parents are off track? There is a major breakdown in the chain, and something is going to go awry. That is the topic of the next section.

SECTION II:
THE ENEMY IN OUR RELATIONSHIPS

Chapter 6

The Root of the War

Before we discuss the specifics of spiritual warfare in the Christian home, we need to gain an understanding of the general context of spiritual warfare, which began with Satan's fall from heaven. We read about Satan's fall in Isaiah:

> All your pomp has been brought down to the grave, along with the noise of your harps; maggots spread out beneath you and worms cover you. How you have fallen from heaven, O morning star, son of the dawn! You have been cast down to the earth, you who once laid low the nations! You said in your heart, "I will ascend to heaven; I will raise my throne above the stars of God; I will sit enthroned on the mount of assembly, on the utmost heights of the sacred mountain. I will ascend above the tops of the clouds; I will make myself like the Most High." (Isaiah 14:11-14)

We clearly see from Isaiah's account that Satan's predominant sin was that he wanted to make himself "like the Most High." Satan wanted to be like God, to rule like God. We also read about Satan's original state as God created him and his fall in Ezekiel 12-17.

> Your heart became proud on account of your beauty, and you corrupted your wisdom because of your splendor (Ezekiel 28:17).

Satan's sin, which caused him to be cast out of heaven, is pride. Essentially, God said to Satan, you want to rule something, rule the earth, or as He refers to it in Isaiah 14:11, "the grave." We also make this inference from the scriptural references to Satan as "the one who is in the world" (1 John 4:4).

Satan, being cast down to earth, made his first appearance to the human race when he came as a serpent to Eve and tempted her to eat the fruit from the tree God forbid Adam and Eve to eat from (Genesis 3:1-5). After God confronted Adam and Eve about their disobedience, He outlined specific consequences first for Satan, then for Eve, and then for Adam. God tells Satan in Genesis 3:15:

> And I will put enmity between you and the woman, and between your offspring and hers.

Here we see the root of spiritual warfare: "enmity between you and the woman." We can infer from God's curse on Satan that although He specifically says "between you and the woman," this is not a curse on woman. Woman has her own consequence she must suffer. Satan's consequence is that while he may rule the earth, he will not do it without enmity. It is not going to be easy for Satan. In fact, there is going to be an ongoing battle.

This battle is between Eve's offspring and Satan's. Does Satan have offspring? Several Scriptures refer to the offspring of Satan. One of these Scriptures is Jesus' own words as recorded in John 8:44: "You belong to your father, the devil, and you want to carry out your father's desire." Satan has offspring of his own; he is a father, in a spiritual sense. Because Satan is an angelic being, he cannot literally reproduce in the flesh (Mark 12:25). However, those who "want to carry out" Satan's desires are, by nature, the children of Satan. In other words, all of us who want to carry out the will of God are God's children. We are the offspring of God's creation of the first man and woman, as created in God's holiness and in perfect relationship with Him. Although we lost that "perfect" relationship, God is loving and forgiving and gave us another chance to regain that relationship through the intercession of His son Jesus Christ. That is why God told Satan in Genesis 3:15: "he will crush your head, and you will strike his heel." The "he" who will crush Satan's head is Jesus. This Genesis account informs us that there will be a war between the offspring of Satan and the offspring of God.

This war is apparent from the first book of the Bible, to the last. In Revelation 12 we read more about this war, which is still being battled:

> When the dragon [Satan] saw that he had been hurled to the earth, he pursued the woman who had given birth to the male child. . . . But the earth helped the woman—Then the dragon was enraged at the woman and went off to make war against the rest of her offspring—those who obey God's commandments and hold to the testimony of Jesus (Revelation 12:13, 16, 17).

Although Satan's head was crushed the moment Jesus gave His last breath nailed to a cross on the hill of Calvary, we are still experiencing the consequence of the original sin, as well as the spiritual battle between the forces. It is because the war has already been won that Satan is "enraged," and still roams the earth. This is evidenced in the daily, monthly, and yearly battles we fight. This is what we refer to as spiritual warfare. Until the Lord returns to set the world straight, we will continue to be caught in the midst of this spiritual war.

Chapter 7

Satan's Plan: Spiritual Warfare on the Homefront

In the ordinary realm of spiritual warfare, we see how God's curse on the genders has affected how men and women relate to one another. We are not going to address the curse on Adam in detail here because it does not directly relate to this discussion. We must note generally, however, that man's curse is twofold and includes not only hard labor on earth, but also physical death. God's curse on woman is not only relevant to spiritual warfare, it is fundamental to woman's relationship to man. In Genesis 3:16 God tells Eve that not only will her pain in childbirth greatly increase, but that:

> Your desire will be for your husband, and he will rule over you.

That statement enlightens the reasons why women struggle to fulfill their marital role as God designed it. It may also bear some spiritual implications for the dynamics found among women who are abusive to men, and speaks directly to the right-wing feminist movement in our country. Think about that verse for a moment: "your desire will be for your husband." Desire is the key word here. Desire in itself is not a bad emotion. In fact, our desires are what make life colorful, and passion, being bred from desire, is the substance that drives us. It is hard to conceive of desire being Eve's curse.

This is especially true when we look at the second part of the verse: "he will rule over you." That in itself is not necessarily a curse either, as God created Eve, or woman, to naturally be in sub-mission to man. The curse is in Eve's desire, followed by her eter-nal earthly inability to fulfill that desire. Have you ever wanted something so much that the desire for it consumed you? You be-came obsessed with it, and could not stop thinking about it or ways to get it? No matter how hard you tried, however, you just could not have it. That, indeed, is a curse. I do not think God was refer-ring to Eve's sexual desire for her husband. Obviously, the sexual relationship between man and woman continues to be a blessing when it falls under the holiness of marriage. What God seemed to be implying is that Eve's desire would be to have her husband's position of authority. Woman, because of her original sin, would spend the rest of her time on earth engaged in an internal struggle between wanting to rule over man and never being able to, result-ing in perpetual frustration. We have seen more evidence of this in the last century. We call it "women's rights." We call it "femi-nism." These movements are not necessarily bad. Indeed, women have been enslaved for thousands of years.

As Christians, we acknowledge that Jesus came to free all people, including women. Historically, Christianity itself freed women in a manner they had never experienced. For instance, Peter wrote in 1 Peter 3:7b: women are "heirs with you [men] of the gracious gift of life." However, not until Jesus comes again to set the world straight will woman be completely free from the internal effects of this curse. In other words, no matter how much power, authority, or even equal status women gain, they will not be satisfied. Women desperately want to be free from this curse, and in this des-peration they struggle.

The point here is not that men rule over women, but that dishar-mony exists between man and woman because of this hierarchy. Furthermore, this disharmony is not because man rules, but be-cause woman wants to. In a commentary on the Genesis 3:16 ac-count, Matthew Henry (2000) writes: "This sentence amounts only to that command, Wives, be in subjection to your own hus-bands; but the entrance of sin has made that duty a punishment, which otherwise it would not have been. If man had not sinned, he would always have ruled with wisdom and love; and, if the woman had not sinned, she would always have obeyed with humility and meekness; and then the dominion would have been no grievance: but our own sin and folly make our yoke heavy" (p. 14).

This curse not only affects women as a gender, but also as individuals in their relationships with men. Christian wives, girlfriends, sisters, and mothers struggle with submission to men. Even the most godly men can be difficult to submit to. Women simply do not want to be ruled by men! And, as we read in the first few chapters of this book, there is no justification for a wife not to be in submission to her godly husband. Although not easy, God provides help through His perfect plan for marriage if it is carried out by both the husband and the wife in utmost faithfulness. However, when one partner is not carrying out God's plan in utmost faithfulness a battleground for spiritual warfare is set.

Before we get into the specifics of spiritual warfare, we must understand first that "internal" spiritual warfare most often happens in homes that are divided, and second that only one of the two people in the marriage are needed to cause division. Jesus warned us in Matthew 12:25:

> Every kingdom divided against itself will be ruined, and every city or *household* divided against itself will not stand (italics added).

In terms of division, if both parties of the relationship are in harmony with God, there is obviously no internal battle to fight. Likewise, when both parties are in disharmony with God, their battles are not necessarily in the "internal" spiritual arena. There may be a spiritual battle they are completely unaware of, but the division in the home is not due to the awareness of spiritual issues. That is not to say that because a husband and wife are both Christians they do not experience spiritual battles, or because a husband and wife are not Christians they do. The clarification comes in the distinction between the "internal" spiritual battle and the "external" spiritual battle. Satan always attempts to penetrate into the "internal" realm, but when a husband and wife are united in Christ, that attempt is often futile because the Holy Spirit is ever present. When a husband

and wife are not Christ-centered, the very nature of the marital relationship is outside of God's plan, and is therefore subject to Satan's plan. Furthermore, when one partner is Christ-centered, and the other is not, an inherent division exists, where one spouse is pitted against the other, and each is backed up by forces of the spiritual realm.

One fundamental fact of spiritual warfare is that Satan does not want what he already has. He wants what he does not have, and his purpose is to thwart directly the advancement of God's will. This also is expressed by Jesus in Matthew 12:26:

If Satan drives out Satan, he is divided against himself.

In non-Christian homes there may be division, but it is often caused by neither person being Christ-centered, and the effects of that spill into all aspects of the unbeliever's life, not just the marriage. The clarification comes in truly understanding that Christian families experience stronger spiritual attacks because they are Christian, but they also have the forces of God helping them withstand these attacks. From a larger spiritual perspective, we see Satan's disruption to marriage, whether Christian or non-Christian, in rising divorce rates. This subtle undermining of the sanctity of marriage has led to a redefining of "family" in our country. No doubt that this is a direct aspect of spiritual warfare in a broader sense but, as stated earlier, Satan does not want the soul that is already his; he wants the one that belongs to God. Herein lies the personalization of the spiritual warfare we may experience.

It is in this personal experience that domestic violence falls. Specific discussion on the dynamics of domestic violence in the Christian home will follow in the next section but, for now, we need to understand that domestic violence is almost unheard of in homes where both husband and wife are in subjection to God. Again, that is not to say that the Christian family does not experience arguments or spiritual attacks. A spiritual battle for Christ-centered families is fought with the husband as the Commanding General, so to speak, with God at the top of his chain of command. The husband's sole purpose is to carry out the mission of God.

Contrast that with the family in which only one partner is a Christian. In that family the spiritual battle does not consist of two people on the same side, but two people living in the same house on opposite sides. Two people are trying to be Commanding Generals, but each is driven by forces in opposition. Jesus said in Matthew 10:34-36:

> Do not suppose that I have come to bring peace to the earth. I did not come to bring peace, but a sword. For I have come to turn a man against his father, a daughter against her mother, a daughter-in-law against her mother-in-law—a man's enemies will be the members of his own household.

When Jesus said this He probably was not referring to all households. He probably was referring to families that are divided. It is interesting to note that this division is caused by a sword. Remember our discussion on parental discipline. The sword of God is His word (Ephesians 6:17). Furthermore, note that Jesus expresses almost all familial relationships here, except the most personal, which is the husband-wife relationship.

Jesus was actually quoting from Micah 7:6. Jesus often quoted the Old Testament and He often clarified Old Testament Scriptures by elaborating, challenging, contrasting, or giving example through parable. He did not do that here, at least not in reference to specific familial relationships. We may presume that Jesus assumed that if one spouse is godly, the other would be also ("Do not be yoked together with unbelievers" 2 Corinthians 6:14). This principle refers to our initial discussion on God's perfect design for marriage. There are a variety of different reasons why a marriage or relationship does not operate entirely within God's design, and God addresses a couple of those in His word. We will save that discussion for later to keep it in a more suitable context. For now, let us just assume that Jesus' admonition about His purpose in bringing the sword of God is relevant to the husband-wife relationship. With that in mind, let us turn to a more specific discussion on Satan's character and strategy in spiritual warfare.

Chapter 8

Satan's Strategies, Character, and Nature

Now that we have a clearer picture of how and why spiritual warfare occurs, let us look at some of the ways that Satan operates within our homes. The best way to do this is through a close examination of the character and behavior of Satan. Let's start by understanding the different names and references made of Satan.

His common name is "Satan" from the Hebrew *satan* and the Greek word *satanas,* literally meaning "adversary." He is referred to as Satan sixty-four times in the Scriptures. In fact, Jesus refers to him as Satan when He speaks of Satan's fall from heaven (Luke 10:18). Thus, "Satan" is not only his common name, but the name by which Jesus calls him. He is also referred to as the "devil." Several Scriptures refer to the devil; all of them are in the New Testament. The Greek words that were translated are *diabolos, daimonizomai,* and *daimonion,* and they literally mean "slanderer." The variation in the Greek uses reflect variations in manifestations (i.e., possessed with devils), rather than different interpretations. Satan is also commonly called "Lucifer," translated from the Hebrew *heylel,* which means "son of the morning," or "light bearer." There is only one reference to Satan as *heylel* in the Scriptures, and it is found in Isaiah's account of Satan's fall from heaven (Isaiah 14:12-17). Lucifer is a popular and well-known reference to Satan. He is also referred to by Jesus several times as "Beelzebub." The Greek translation of this reference is "lord of the house." Satan is also referred to once as "Belial" (2 Corinthians 6:15).

The Scriptures also make reference to Satan's character. He has been called "the evil one" (1 John 5:19), "the tempter" (Matthew 4:3, 1 Thessalonians 3:5), "prince of this world" (John 12:31), "god of this age" (2 Corinthians 4:4), "ruler of the kingdom of the air" (Ephesians 2:2), and "accuser of our brothers" in Revelation 12:10. Satan has also been characterized as a spirit being (Ephesians 6:11-12).

Several Scriptures refer to him as a serpent, as well as a dragon. John's vision of our future, as recorded in Revelation 12:7-9, refers to Satan as a "serpent."

> The great dragon was hurled down—that ancient serpent called the devil, or Satan, who leads the whole world astray (Revelation 12:9).

Satan is a creature; however, Satan is also a spirit being. In Ezekiel 28:14 we read that Satan was "anointed as a guardian cherub." Thus, Satan is of the cherubim angels, whose purpose seems to be to guard the holiness of God (Genesis 3:22-24). We also read in Ezekiel that he was the highest of all angelic creatures (Ezekiel 28:12).

We also know from God's word about the personality of Satan. Genesis 3:1 says that the serpent "was more crafty than any of the wild animals," and 2 Corinthians 11:3 says that "Eve was deceived by the serpent's cunning." We read in the book of Job that Satan approaches God and carries on a logical conversation with Him. These accounts tell us that Satan is clearly intelligent. We also know from Ezekiel's account that Satan possesses wisdom (Ezekiel 28:17b). In addition, we read in Revelation 12:17 that "the dragon was enraged at the woman—." We also know he experiences pride (Ezekiel 28:17, Isaiah 14:12-14, 1 Timothy 3:6). So, we can assume that Satan has emotions. Finally, we read in 2 Timothy 2:26 "—the trap of the devil, who has taken them captive to do his will." Thus, Satan has a will of his own.

Now that we know a little more about the character and nature of Satan, let us review Scriptures that give us more specific insights into his strategies. The first account of Satan, as we already discussed, is found in Genesis 3, where Satan tricked Eve. First, he challenged her by asking her to rethink what God told her: "Did God really say?" (Genesis 3:1). Questioning God sometimes challenges our faith and begs our human intellect; this is where Satan often tempts us. Once Eve questioned what God had said, Satan went in for the kill. He lied to her (verse 4). Part of Satan's strategy against us sometimes includes a subtle challenge of our intellect and/or knowledge. He also seems to almost always include some form of lying, whether subtle or blatant. The more knowledgeable we are about God's word, the more subtle Satan is. In fact, as Christians, we must be extremely careful because Jesus warned us that in the "end times" false prophets will come to "deceive even the elect—if that were possible" (Matthew 24:24, Mark 13:22).

Satan lied to Eve, and he lies to us. Jesus confirms Satan's deceit when He says, "When he lies, he speaks his native language, for he is a liar and the father of lies" (John 8:44). Satan continued by tempting Eve. He told Eve that there was a benefit for her to eat the fruit. He held the forbidden fruit in a light that made it seem irresistible. Indeed, temptation is what Satan is notorious for. Even Jesus, being led by the Spirit into the desert, was tempted by Satan (Matthew 4). Satan tempts us to commit acts directly against God's expressed will, and he desires to thwart God's purpose by misleading us. Temptation can come in the form of drinking a beer, picking up a prostitute, cursing, or maybe even buying that pretty house on the hill that you just cannot afford.

Not all temptation is provoked by Satan. In James 1:14 we read: "but each one is tempted when, by his own evil desire, he is dragged away and enticed." Our nature is sinful. On the other hand, Satan knows that our inherent "flaw," if you will, is that sinful nature, and he certainly capitalizes on that. As recorded in 1 Thessalonians 3:5, Paul wrote: "I was afraid that in some way the tempter might have tempted you and our efforts might have been useless." Satan, the tempter, always has a purpose to thwart God's plans; Paul's primary concern was that Satan had achieved his goal through tempting the believers of the Church at Thessalonica.

Another account of Satan's strategic plan at tempting God's children is found in the book of Job. Job suffered immense losses. The purpose for those losses is outlined in the first two chapters of the book. When we read those in the full context, we learn that Job suffered the loss of everything dear to him, and even his own health, because it was God's plan that Satan would tempt Job to "curse you [God] to your face" (Job 1:11). We learn several things from the book of Job about Satan's plan, his nature, and his capability. We learn that Satan can do nothing against those who belong to the Lord, without God's expressed permission first (Luke 22:31). God put conditions on what Satan could do to Job, and Satan followed those conditions. We also learn that Satan has the capability to physically kill us (because Job's servants and children died) and to physically kill animals (Job's flocks were destroyed). In Job we see that Satan accomplished this through other human beings (Job 1:15 and 17), through supernatural forces (Job 1:16), and through natural forces (Job 1:19). Satan's final ploy against Job was to torture him with painful sores. Thus, Satan has the capability to inflict disease.

We must understand that Satan is not always responsible for the death, disease, and loss we experience in life. The comforting news is that when he is responsible, it is only because God has a higher plan. In Job's case, God allowed Satan to wreak havoc in Job's life because God knew Job would pass the "test." That test was initiated by Satan's accusation that Job would "curse God." Accusation is another one of Satan's strategies. Revelation 12:10b verifies this: "For the accuser of our brothers, who accuses them before our God day and night—." Satan is a finger-pointer. He demeans and demoralizes us day and night. In Job's case, Satan's finger-pointing led to a challenge. Satan tempted Job to fail, and do exactly what Satan accused him of doing.

We also see Satan using temptation in the book of Matthew (Chapter 4), where Satan appeared to Jesus in the desert. From this account of Jesus' temptation we see that Satan attempted to deceive Jesus. On some level it is comforting to know that even the Son of God fell under temptation. Not only did Satan attempt to deceive Jesus, he used Scripture against Jesus. This is very important because it tells us that Satan knows Scripture, and knows how to use it against us. He is intimately familiar with it, and his subtle deception of the Christian people generally comes through the twisting of the word we value so much. Indeed, for Christians, the word is our road map of life, and it is an obvious warfare strategy for Satan to attempt to lead us astray through the subtle turning of the map. Read Matthew Chapter 4, if you have not already, to understand how Satan attempts to use our own sword against us. This is a crucial understanding in the arena of spiritual warfare. The more we know about Satan's strategies, the better equipped we are for the onslaught of spiritual attacks we face.

Another strategy Satan uses in warfare is to counterfeit God. We see this strategy throughout the Bible. Remember, Satan's expulsion from heaven was because of his pride and his desire to be "like the Most High" (Isaiah 14:14). The first obvious account of Satan's manifestation of his pride is found in the book of Exodus. There, God's word reveals to us Satan's true ability to counterfeit God. God had sent Moses and Aaron before the Pharaoh of Egypt to warn Egypt to let God's people, who had been enslaved in Egypt, go. God also instructed Moses and Aaron that He would help them perform a miracle before Pharaoh. That is exactly what Moses and Aaron did. Then Pharaoh "summoned wise men and sorcerers and the Egyptian magicians also did the same things by their secret arts: Each one threw down his staff and it became a snake" (Exodus 7:11-12). So, here we have a battle between men of God, and men of Satan. Moses and Aaron's challenge was matched in turning the water of Egypt into blood (Exodus 7:22). The Egyptian magicians also were able to counterfeit God's plague of frogs (Exodus 8:7). When it came to God's other plagues, however, Satan was no match for God. Finally, in verse 19 of Chapter 8, the magicians said to Pharaoh, "This is the finger of God." Satan was defeated. From this biblical account, we see again that Satan has limitations. He always will because he is not God. More important, we see that he has a tremendous amount of power, and is quite capable of deceiving us through his counterfeiting strategies.

Jesus also spoke of Satan's ability to counterfeit God. In Matthew 24:24 it is recorded, "For false Christs and false prophets will appear and perform great signs and miracles to deceive even the elect—if that were possible." The book of Revelation also recorded, referring to Satan: "[He] made the earth and its inhabitants worship the beast, *whose fatal wound had been healed.* And he performed great and miraculous signs, even causing fire to come down from heaven to earth in full view of men" (Revelation 13:12 and 13, italics added). Perhaps the most intriguing aspect of Satan's warfare strategy is that he even counterfeits the Holy Trinity of God. To the Christian, God represents three aspects in one embodiment: God, the Father; Jesus, the Son; and the Holy Spirit, which all Christians possess. In Revelation we read about the dragon (Satan as the head), the anti-Christ (the son of Satan), and the false prophet (the false spirit who gives testimony against Jesus) (see Revelation 19:10e). To anyone who is not intimately familiar with God, Satan's brand of counterfeit can seem very real.

Another strategy Satan uses, which is perhaps even more crucial to our understanding of spiritual warfare, is division. Anyone who has been in the military will tell you that if you can cause division in the ranks of your opponent, you virtually render them completely immobile. They become their own enemies. Jesus said: "Every kingdom divided against itself will be ruined, and every city or household divided against itself will not stand" (Matthew 12:25). As discussed in the last chapter, this particular strategy of Satan is at the root of the personal spiritual warfare we may face in our own homes.

So, we know from biblical accounts that Satan is a liar, a tempter, an accuser, and a murderer. He attempts to execute these strategies through the spreading of false doctrine, through actual meddling in our lives, through physical attacks, and through mental attacks. However, Satan does not merely take these actions, he does so with great fierceness and an undying motivation. We are warned in 1 Peter 5:8: "Your enemy the devil prowls around like a roaring lion looking for someone to devour." Indeed he does. If that has not become evident to you already, maybe some facts about domestic violence will convince you of the reality of Satan's fierceness.

SECTION III:
MANIFESTATIONS OF DEMONIC INFLUENCE: THE HARD TRUTH ABOUT FAMILY VIOLENCE

Chapter 9

Some Facts About Domestic Violence: Till Death Do Us Part?

The National Crime Victimization Survey (NCVS), sponsored by the U.S. Department of Justice (DOJ), is given annually to approximately 50,000 households and 100,000 individuals in the United States. The NCVS is a paper and pencil survey that asks respondents about crimes they have experienced within a certain time frame. The NCVS has recently been redesigned to address the academic criticisms about its design. A newer method by which domestic violence data is gathered is the National Violence Against Women Survey (NVAWS), sponsored by the joint effort of the National Institute of Justice (NIJ) and the Centers for Disease Control and Prevention (CDC). Another method for determining national crime information is through the Uniform Crime Reports (UCR), which is sponsored by the Federal Bureau of Investigation (FBI).

All methods are commonly used to address crime (and particularly domestic violence) on a national level; however, the NCVS is respected more than the UCR as an accurate reflection of domestic violence. This is because the UCR is a compilation of police reports from various police agencies throughout the country. It is a well-known fact that domestic violence is a "hidden crime," and is grossly underreported to the police. Less than 55 percent of the respondents to the NCVS claimed that they reported their assault to the police. The UCR reflects only reports to the police, and does not reveal much detail about the crime, the circumstances of the crime, or until recently, the victim-offender relationship. The NCVS is a self-report measure of crime victimization. This means that it is not based on reports to the police. The NCVS attempts to capture the actual prevalence and circumstances of victimization in this country by directly asking victims about their experiences, regardless of whether they reported those experiences to the police. In addition, the nature of the crime is more specifically addressed in the NCVS so that more details about domestic violence can be determined.

As of the writing of this book, the most recent and complete NCVS report was in 1992-1993 (Bachman and Saltzman, 1995). The NVAWS has been reported on more recently, occurring in 1995-1996 (Tjaden, 1997). Although they are similar surveys, unless otherwise noted, all discussion will be based on the NCVS. Although the data is not recent, the 1992-1993 NCVS reveals much about domestic violence in this country.

Broadly, the NCVS reveals that every year almost 5 million females age twelve and older sustain violent victimizations. Although the NCVS does not survey 5 million women, its respondents theoretically represent an "average" sample of the population in this country. Taking the prevalence rates from this large sample of individuals, researchers then extrapolate them into national rates based on the country's entire population.

This research reveals that nearly 75 percent of women who are violently victimized experienced lone-offender victimizations. In other words, only one perpetrator participated in the crime. Of the 75 percent of female victims of single perpetrators, 29 percent reported that the perpetrator was an intimate. The NCVS defines an intimate as a husband, ex-husband, boyfriend, or ex-boyfriend. That is a staggering statistic. *Nearly 30 percent of women who report violent victimization report that the perpetrator was someone they were intimate with.*

These statistics are tragic on a national level, but when we bring it to the level of our neighborhoods, our schools, our churches, and our own homes, we should be very alarmed. You may think that your community, or at least your church, is immune to the problem, but research estimates that *two in every twenty-five people have been physically abused by a spouse or other intimate partner.* If you are one of those people, you know all too well about the prevalence of domestic violence. Indeed, the NCVS is not merely a national victimization survey, but a painful reality in your own life.

The NCVS reveals that *of the 29 percent of female victims of intimates, 9 percent reported the perpetrator to be a spouse, 4 percent an ex-spouse, and 16 percent a boyfriend or ex-boyfriend.* Because the research report does not separate the boyfriend and ex-boyfriend categories, we cannot determine which relationship type occurs most frequently in violent victimizations. Although this information may be important in terms of spiritual ramifications, the general point is that women are being violently victimized by men they love or once loved.

What about male victims? Men rarely report their victimizations to the police. Although the NCVS attempts to circumvent this dilemma, we must acknowledge that men may hesitate even to self-report domestic violence because of the perception equating victimization with weakness. Weakness is a socially forbidden characteristic for a man to demonstrate. So, when we learn that 4 percent of male victims report their perpetrator to be an intimate, we must consider that this may not be an accurate statistic. We must acknowledge from these figures that *women are almost six times more likely than men to experience violence by an intimate.*

Of women who experience violence by men they love, 1 percent report that violence to be rape or sexual assault. *Of all rapes and sexual assaults reported by women, 26 percent were committed by an intimate.* Therefore, rape is not the most common form of intimate abuse, but more than a quarter of all rapes in this country are committed by an intimate. In 1992, 500,000 rapes and sexual assaults were reported to NCVS interviewers. Over half of these rapes or sexual assaults were committed by a friend or acquaintance of the victim. That translates to *over 250,000 rapes and sexual assaults perpetrated by a known assailant.* Again, keep in mind that reported rates are just that. None of these figures speak to the "hidden" crimes that go unreported.

One and a half percent of women who report violence by an intimate report that violence to be an aggravated assault, and over 6 percent report it to be simple assault. Simple assault has been defined as "an attack without a weapon resulting either in minor injury (that is, bruises, black eyes, cuts, scratches, or swelling) or in un-determined injury requiring less than two days hospitalization. It also includes attempted assault without a weapon and verbal threats of assault" (Bachman and Saltzman, 1995, p. 3). Aggravated assault has been defined as "an attack or attempted attack with a weapon regardless of whether an injury occurred as well as an attack without a weapon when serious injury results. Serious injury includes broken bones, loss of teeth, internal injuries, loss of consciousness, and any injury requiring two or more days of hospitalization" (p. 3). Even though these numbers seem low, consider that *52 percent of women reporting a violent victimization by an intimate reported that they sustained injuries as a result of the victimization, and 41 percent reported that they received injuries that required medical care.* Imagine being intentionally physically injured by someone you love. For some women, their worst imaginations became reality. Because we are discussing a subgroup of victims, these statistics may not seem impressive, but consider that *female victims of violence by an intimate are more often injured by the violence than females victimized by a stranger.*

Not only are women injured more often by men they love than by strangers, but a large number of these men use weapons. Of those victims who reported that a weapon was involved in their victimization, *18 percent were involved in an intimate relationship with their perpetrator.*

Even more frightening is the fact that these men may kill their victims. According to the UCR, in 1992, 28.3 percent of all female homicides (in which the relationship of the offender was identi-fied) were committed by an intimate (FBI, 1992). In other words, *almost 30 percent of all females murdered in this country are murdered by someone they love.* Contrast that with the UCR finding that 3.6 percent of all male homicide victims are killed by an inti-mate. Also, keep in mind that in 31 percent of female homicides the victim-offender relationship was not identified. So, the per-centage may be even greater. These numbers are based on police reported homicides, not missing persons.

Through this picture painted by the NCVS and UCR, we can conclude that our fear of crime may be misdirected. It is not dark alleyways we need to fear as much as it is our own homes. Women all over this country are arming themselves, carrying pepper spray, learning defense and safety tactics, but no one has told them that they need to be on guard when they come home. Why don't women just leave their abusers? Good question! We will discuss that in more detail in the next chapter, but in terms of statistics, evidence points to one major reason.

Why Do Women Stay in Abusive Relationships?

The fundamental reason a Christian woman may stay in an abusive relationship is tied to her spirituality and the church's response. A study done by Jim Alsdurf (cited in Grady, 2001, pp. 40-44) revealed that of 5,700 Protestant pastors surveyed, 26 percent said they "normally tell a woman being abused that she should continue to submit, and trust God would honor her action by either stopping the abuse or giving her the strength to endure it." Almost 25 percent of pastors said a lack of the wife's submissiveness is what caused the abuse. A majority of the pastors responded that "it is better for a woman to tolerate some level of violence in the home—even though it is not God's perfect will—than to seek separation that might end in divorce." Seventy-one percent said they would never advise an abused woman to leave her husband, and 92 percent said they would never counsel an abused woman to seek a divorce. This is the type of counsel that keeps an abused woman in bondage, and perpetuates her faulty sense of marital obligation and Christian duty. Another reason women remain in abusive relationships is fear, whether founded or not, of further retaliation by the abuser. The NCVS reveals that the victimization rate of women separated from their husbands is about three times higher than that of divorced women, and twenty-five times higher than that of married women. From these statistics we can assume that when a woman attempts to separate herself from her abusive husband, she is at the highest risk for physical violence.

The NVAWS collected national-level data on the crime of stalking. Stalking includes such behavior as making overt threats, making death threats, spying on the victim, and vandalizing the victim's property. A report on the NVAWS reveals that about 1.4

million people a year are victims of stalking (Tjaden, 1997). Of all people surveyed by the NVAWS, 8 percent of women and 2 percent of men said they had been stalked in their lifetime. Of all stalking victims in this survey, about 80 percent were women. *The projected rate of total female stalking victims is 8.2 million.* Furthermore, "the survey showed that stalking was strongly linked to the controlling behavior and physical, emotional, and sexual abuse perpetrated against women by intimate partners" (p. 1). Less than one-half of all female stalking victims claimed they had reported their victimization to the police. Again, we see an underreporting trend, meaning that stalking may be a bigger problem than these statistics reveal.

Episodes of stalking tend to last less than a year, but a few individuals reported that it continued for more than five years. Of all stalkers, only 21 percent of women reported their stalker to be a stranger. In contrast, almost 80 percent of stalkers stalk women they know. Men, on the other hand, are significantly more likely to be stalked by a stranger. Furthermore, *approximately 50 percent of female stalking victims were stalked by an intimate partner. Of these women, almost 80 percent reported that at some point in their relationship with the perpetrator they had been physically assaulted by him.* This clearly tells us that women who are abused by the men they love continue to suffer the abuse even after they flee the relationship.

Why don't these women file a restraining order against him? The NVAWS revealed that 80 percent of women who received a restraining order reported that the order was violated. At that point, the issue is no longer how an abused woman can stop the abuse, but what the justice system will or will not do to protect her. Sadly, only 15 percent of female stalking victims reported that the stalking stopped because of police involvement.

Taken as a whole, these statistics imply that domestic violence is a devastating and often deadly problem. Although one may read these statistics and walk away in disbelief, we must keep in perspective what constitutes domestic violence. We often assume that domestic violence occurs only when a woman receives a severe beating. Indeed, even the data from the UCR, NCVS, and the NVAWS tends to gravitate toward the mid to upper "range" of the violence spectrum. In the next chapter we will discuss the specific varieties of abuse.

Chapter 10

The Five Types of Abuse

When we think of family abuse we may be tempted to catego-rize the types of abuse in a least-to-most severity scale. In other words, we may want to place verbal abuse at the left end of the spectrum, and place physical abuse at the right end. That view minimizes certain types of abuse. For example, you may think that being called a vulgar name is not as bad as being hit, or even more faulty, that being called a vulgar name does not even constitute an act of domestic violence. This chapter is intended to expose that lie, and discuss the dynamics involved in the abusive spouse's con-tinuance of violence.

Verbal/Emotional Abuse

Verbal and emotional abuse has been occurring since the begin-ning of man's presence on earth. Indeed, God Himself warns us about our tongues throughout the Bible. He says: "Consider what a great forest is set on fire by a small spark. The tongue also is a fire, a world of evil among the parts of the body. It corrupts the whole person, sets the whole course of his life on fire, and is itself set on fire by hell. All kinds of animals, birds, reptiles, and crea-tures of the sea are being tamed and have been tamed by man, but no man can tame the tongue. It is a restless evil, full of deadly poi-son" (James 3:5-8).

The most interesting aspect of these verses is that God is warn-ing us of the serious damage that can occur from one small spark. In and of itself verbal abuse does not seem that bad, but slowly and over time, it chips away at the victim's sense of self, functional concept of self, and undermines faith. Imagine being told that you are fat, day after day; "lose weight," "you make me sick," "all you do is eat," "all I have to do is slap her thigh and ride the wave in." Some people laugh about these comments as if they are part of a juvenile game. "You're so dumb," "what a blonde," "you'd forget your head if it wasn't attached." Even if said jokingly, these kinds of statements can hurt. They are words that can devastate the human spirit. God knows that. We also have to acknowledge that women who are abusive to their husbands are most often abusive in the areas of verbal and emotional abuse. Proverbs 19:13b compares a "quarrelsome wife" to a "constant dripping." Not only can argumentativeness be annoying, it can be hurtful and damaging.

Perhaps just as damaging is emotional abuse. Verbal abuse can be blatant and easy to recognize; emotional abuse can be much more subtle. Emotional abuse includes behaviors such as playing "mind games," convincing her that she is crazy, mentally unstable, or sick, and making her feel guilty. Abusive men often accuse their partners of having an affair. Abusers are often extremely jealous and insecure, and they tend to project that onto their victims. "Where were you?" "Why did it take you twenty minutes to drive home?" "I know you had someone over while I was gone." These types of statements, to an outside observer, may not seem abusive at all, but the woman who lives with these constant inferences of guilt may begin to feel guilty. She may feel as if she must rush home, and may even stop going out because of the repercussions when she returns home. Another form of emotional abuse shows itself in the family's finances. An abuser may make her ask for money, may take money away from her, may prevent her from working because of jealousy and fear of losing control over her, or may force her to work to "pay her own way," not being willing to take any financial responsibility for her. He may even refuse to pay any and all bills that are in her name, or may force her to put all the bills in her name so he will not destroy his own credit generally. He treats her unequally in the financial realm.

Other forms of emotional abuse occur when the abuser treats his partner like a servant, or makes comments such as "I'm the king of the castle," or "captain of the ship." Referring to our discussion on family roles for a moment, we must keep in mind that we are not discussing the roles of headship and submission, but discussing using male privilege to control and manipulate women. Making an important decision as the man of the family, after having prayed with his wife about it, is different from saying "get up and get me something to eat" in a demanding and demeaning manner. Sadly, many young men believe that women are subservient. Even sadder, many young Christian men stumble upon the Ephesians and Colossians verses we discussed at the beginning of the book, and use them to justify their continued abuse toward their partners.

Another form of emotional abuse is when abusers make threats of a various nature. He may threaten to take the children if she ever leaves. He may threaten to commit suicide if she leaves. He may even threaten to have her arrested or committed to a psychiatric hospital.

An even more subtle form of emotional abuse comes from the misuse of privileged information. In a husband-wife relationship an unparalleled emotional intimacy typically exists. They have told each other secrets that they have told no other person. They know each other so well that their vulnerabilities and sensitivities have been left bare on occasion. They have laughed together and cried together. Even in abusive relationships, a certain aspect of marriage, perhaps a sanctity from God, makes it a sacred ground where no one else can tread. When an abuser decides he wants to "get to her," or "show her," he may use as a threat those secrets she has shared, or may attack her in her most vulnerable spot. For example, imagine if you told your spouse, in a moment of intimacy, that you felt guilty for the accidental death of your sibling when you were a child. Later your spouse, in the heat of an argument, says, "You just wish me dead like you did to your own brother."

Whether it is being called a name, being referred to in a derogatory manner, or constantly being accused of something, these behaviors are destructive. They leave the kinds of bruises that require much more healing than bruises of the physical nature. They penetrate hearts and scar souls. If you live with this behavior, know that God sees and hears, and Jesus weeps over your pain. If you do not live with this type of behavior from someone you love, pray and ask God to give you compassion and understanding for those who do. Imagine what it is like, and next time someone shares with you about the pain of being treated so harshly by someone she loves, do not treat her as her partner does, but as Jesus would. Say to her what you think Jesus would say.

Physical/Sexual Abuse

Physical abuse is also mentioned in the Bible. Malachi 2:10-16 speakes on marriage and divorce. We will look at this again when we discuss divorce, but for now, pay particular attention to verse 16:

> "I hate divorce," says the Lord God of Israel, "and I hate a man's covering himself with violence as well as with his garment," says the Lord Almighty (Malachi 2:16).

As with all of God's words, it seems more than mere coincidence that He speaks of divorce in the same context as He speaks of violence. The Israelites had divorced the wives of their youth, thus being abusive to them, taking foreign wives instead. One interpretation of this passage is taken from a commentary by Matthew Henry (1991): "In all this they covered violence with their garment; they abused their wives, and were vexatious to them, and yet, in the sight of others, they pretended to be very loving to them and tender of them, and to cast a skirt over them. It is common for those who do violence to advance some specious pretense or other wherewith to cover it as with a garment" (p. 1600). Henry is implying that our "covering" ourselves, as Adam and Eve first did in Eden, is detestable to God, whether it is our flesh or our sins we are trying to cover. When God said, "I hate a man's covering himself with violence as well as with his garment," He literally meant that. While some theologians question whether the Israelites were physically violent toward their wives, Malachi 2:14-16 reveals that they were abusive in some manner. The point in this Scripture is that violence between a man and his wife is not new. That, too, has been going on for centuries, and God specifically says He hates it.

Many men may say to themselves, "I'm really not abusive because I never have or never would hit my wife." Many wives may
say the same thing. However, as with verbal and emotional abuse,
much more is involved in physical abuse than leaving bruises.
Even the threat of physical intimidation constitutes abuse. A husband looks at his wife, or makes gestures toward her that make her
afraid he will hurt her, even if he never does. That is violence.
He may be so angry that he has "murder in his eyes." That is abuse.
He may smack his open hand with his closed fist as if to gesture
that he may hit her. Even if he never touches her, that is abuse. He
may circle around her, or get extremely close to her face. He may
become so irate that his entire face is red, his blood vessels pro-
trude, and saliva flies out of his mouth. That is abuse. Being afraid
that your spouse will physically hurt you is abuse.

Another act of physical intimidation that does not require direct
physical contact occurs when a partner smashes or throws objects,
and intentionally destroys the other partner's property. For instance, he may say "you make me so mad," while he is intentionally stepping on something to break it. Maybe he throws things at
her. Maybe he throws things in the opposite direction. Either way
it is physically threatening and emotionally frightening to consider that he can completely lose control.

Yet another tactic that an abusive partner may use to intimidate
is to abuse the family pets. An old quip says that when you have a
bad day you come home and kick the dog. Or maybe throw the cat.
Some people actually do that. In fact, many victims of stalking report that the stalker killed their pet. A fine line exists between
harming an animal and harming a person. It may be so fine that
crossing over it is as inevitable as blinking an eye.

The more obvious forms of physical abuse consist of making threats to hurt someone, displaying a weapon, and actually
making physical contact. Physical abuse is frightening, but even
threatening to hurt someone may invoke fear. Some abusers make
threats toward their partners in a joking manner. Violence is never
to be joked about. Some abusers are not joking, but make good on
their threats. Imagine a man coming at his wife with all of his
weight and strength, and she knows that she is about to be battered.

This happens to thousands of women. Story after story is reported of women who have been beaten, stabbed, choked, kicked, slapped, pushed, and punched by their partners. A woman received a broken knee from being hit over and over with a broom handle. Another blacked out when she fell to the floor after being choked into unconsciousness. Still another received a black eye when she was pulled off the couch and kicked in the face while she lay on the floor. One received a concussion when her head was repeatedly beat into the wall. A broken back resulted from being kicked on the spine several times. A victim received a broken arm from being grabbed as she tried to flee her enraged husband. You may be appalled to hear that these tragedies actually happen. Even more appalling is that they occur at the hands of people who are supposed to love and protect the very women they are abusing.

Sexual abuse is one of the most misunderstood forms of family abuse, a misunderstanding resulting from the idea that a man cannot rape his wife. Indeed, rape itself is not a new phenomenon; we read about sexual abuse in the Bible. The first record is the rape of Dinah in Genesis 34. Shechem did not actually rape Dinah in the sense we tend to think of rape because the Bible says "his heart was drawn" to her and "he loved the girl and spoke tenderly to her" (Genesis 34:3). Shechem had feelings for Dinah. Was that rape? The Bible tells us nothing about Dinah's feelings for Shechem. We can only assume they were merely acquaintances before having sex because in the verse prior it says he saw her and then violated her (Genesis 34:2). Then, his feelings for her follow. We can assume Dinah was not too pleased about Shechem simply because it says nothing about how Dinah felt. Perhaps she was neutral about the situation; but, more likely, Dinah was very upset. Shechem was a foreigner and the Israelites did not believe in premarital sex (Genesis 34:7). Her relations with Shechem filled her family with "grief and fury" (Genesis 34:7). This story may be the equivalent to a modern day date rape situation.

Another biblical account of sexual abuse is found in 2 Samuel 13:1-22. This is an incestual rape. We also read about the violent rape of the Levite's concubine in Judges 19:25 and 20:5. She died from this attack. Several other places within the Bible tell about the sexual promiscuity and immorality of mankind. It is perhaps the most written about form of abuse. Very little, however, is actually said about marital rape. In fact, the only mention is:

> The wife's body does not belong to her alone but also to her husband. In the same way, the husband's body does not belong to him alone but to his wife. Do not deprive each other except by mutual consent and for a time, so that you may devote yourselves to prayer (1 Corinthians 7:4-5a).

Some may read this and say to their spouse, "See? Your body is mine to do with what I want, so you have to do what I say." Perhaps someone has said that to you. Notice the very important clause Paul gives here: *mutual consent.* When we read the entire chapter in context, Paul is clearly saying not to sexually deprive each other because to do so can lead to the temptation to commit adultery due to our lack of self-control. In other words, if we want sex that much, we should get it from each other so that we are not tempted to get it elsewhere. Notice Paul was cautious in his instruction. In verse 6 he wrote: "I say this as a concession, not as a command" (1 Corinthians 7:6).

We must be careful here too, because sexual abuse can occur in the form of guilt: "If you will not do it, I'll find someone who will." Making your spouse feel guilty for not wanting to participate in a particular sexual act, or for not wanting to have sex in general is emotional manipulation. It is sexual abuse.

Another form of sexual abuse is demonstrated through groping and sexually demeaning attitudes. The difference between an enjoyed mutual sexual experience between a husband and wife, and an unwanted and unsolicited sexual confrontation is the difference between feeling blessed and feeling violated. Sometimes, feelings indicate whether abuse is taking place, because what one person experiences as pleasurable, another may experience as a violation. Either way, when a spouse is aware of the sexual likes and dislikes of his or her partner, but continues to focus on the dislikes, overtones of sexual abuse exist. For example, a man walks up behind his wife while she is doing the dishes and firmly grabs her breasts;

one woman finds that to be a sign that she is desirable to him, another thinks that she is merely a sex object to him. In the subtle arena of sexual signals, communication is essential to understanding each other. The difference between an abusive relationship and a healthy relationship is respect. Anytime a husband causes his wife to feel that she is only a sexual object to him is sexual abuse.

An even more blatant form of abuse is outright sexual force. Again, it may be difficult to believe that rape occurs within a marriage, but it does. Rape in marriage occurs mainly because of a false idea that women are property; once she is married she is owned and ruled. Remember our initial discussion on the roles of marriage. Wives are equal "heirs of the gracious gift of life" (1 Peter 3:7). They are not property. As with stranger rape, marital rape occurs when the wife is forced against her will to participate in a sexual act. Stories include women who have had pillows placed over their faces while they were forced to have sex; women whose hair was pulled as they were told to shut up and perform fellatio on their husbands; women who were tied down as they were forced to have anal sex; and women expected to perform sexual acts similar to ones seen in pornographic movies. Even though these acts occur between a husband and a wife, they are still rape.

Spiritual Abuse: Alicia's Story

Spiritual abuse is perhaps the most harmful form of abuse. All abuse causes damage to the spirit, so all abuse can be considered spiritual abuse. Spiritual abuse needs to be recognized as a separate form because it has its own distinct characteristics. Sadly, spiritual abuse is the least addressed type of abuse, but for the Christian family, is the most damaging. This factual vignette gives heartbreaking testimony to the reality of spiritual abuse.

Alicia married Doug twenty years ago. She was in her late twenties and he was in his thirties when they married. Both of them were Christians. Doug's abusive behavior began almost immediately, as most abusive behavior does, with verbal abuse. Criticisms and put-downs quickly became a daily part of their relationship. Alicia struggled through it, accepting Doug's behavior toward her as a "normal" part of their marriage. Alicia reports that Doug physically abused her very rarely, about once a year. The relationship went from bad to worse several years into their marriage when Doug started using drugs. Doug's drug use brought the physical, psychological, and spiritual effects of addiction, and his behavior not only intensified, it became blatantly spiritual. Doug began telling Alicia "a wife should be submissive to her husband." He told her that she was the "wife of Satan," and at other times that she was Mary Magdalene. He called her a whore. He locked her in the bedroom for days at a time, telling her she was too evil to talk to, or to touch the children they had together.

Doug's abusive behavior escalated, and he began to experience what psychiatrists call "drug-induced psychosis." He was convinced that Alicia was having an affair, and took drastic measures against her. When they went into a store together, Doug made her walk ten feet ahead of him, with her head down and covered, and if she looked up or spoke to anyone, she would be beaten when they returned home. Even worse, Alicia says, Doug was convinced that men were having sex with her at night when she and Doug were in bed together. He was hallucinating, and took it out on Alicia by forcing her to wear a sock in her vagina so no one could penetrate her. Due to Doug's delusional thinking, coupled with his religious beliefs, his abuse took on an even more spiritual, but demonic, nature.

On many occasions, Alicia reports, her husband would force her to get down on her hands and knees at his feet, with her head covered, as she prayed for forgiveness. He would sometimes keep her awake for three or four days at a time "preaching" to her from the Bible. Alicia reflects that much of what Doug said was twisted and against what the Bible actually says. She endured his tyrannical behavior, because if she questioned what he said or believed, the consequence would be corporal punishment. Doug believed that women should be silent and submissive. He also believed that he was the head of her, and Christ was the head of him.

Who can argue with that? Does not God's word say that? At the same time, however, Doug was beating his wife and using the Bible to justify it. We will discuss this in more detail in the chapter on demonic possession. For now, we can acknowledge Alicia's story and the serious spiritual implications in Doug's abuse. Not only did Doug become paranoid and hallucinate, he also became extreme and fanatical in his religious beliefs. Alicia reports that he would even write Scriptures on the walls of their home, using markers. These Scriptures were either from the book of Revelation, or the Ephesians and Colossians verses referring to submissiveness of the wife.

Alicia, finally to the point where she could not take any more abuse, left Doug and entered a battered women's shelter. When she arrived at the shelter, her chest was bruised, and she was emotionally confused. During her stay at the shelter, she and the children improved their mental conditions, and began the long process of healing the wounds Doug had inflicted. She successfully completed the domestic violence program at the shelter, and moved into a transitional housing program, which was designed to help her and the children get back on their feet both emotionally and financially so they could live free from abuse, and independent of Doug. The outlook was positive for Alicia, but a very deep part of her felt guilty for having left Doug. She had heard him tell her for so many years how evil she was, what a whore, what a sinner, that she felt as if he was right, and that she had abandoned him, and sinned against God. Alicia shares that she felt and still feels that she is the one who had to ask for forgiveness.

Sadly, while in the transitional program, Doug made contact with Alicia and the children. This time, he promised, things would be different if she returned to him. He would quit using drugs, and they could move to another state and start life over. Alicia would not just "give up" several years of marriage. After all, they both agreed that it was God's will for a wife to stay with her husband, despite adversity. So Alicia and the children moved with Doug, away from her familiar surroundings and her family.

Tragically, Doug's "miraculous" change lasted only three months. He started using drugs again, and in a short period of time his abuse began again. This time, his addiction left the family homeless, and they were forced to live in a tent. Alicia had another child with Doug during this time. Alicia shares in an almost matter-of-fact manner that Doug beat her nearly to the point of death. For no apparent reason, as she was nursing the baby, he began to beat her. She says she does not remember much of that time in her life, but that the children have told her what happened. The oldest one had stepped in to stop his father from beating his mother, which in turn caused a physical altercation between them. Alicia, wanting to protect her child, began to fight back for the first time in their marriage. As a result, Doug beat her to near unconsciousness. She says she attempted to crawl out of the tent opening, when he pulled out a gun and threatened to kill her. When she asked him why he was doing this to her, he replied that he never said he was going to kill her, and that she was "crazy." Alicia says she lost consciousness shortly after and that she was bleeding from her ears. Doug had also hit her in the throat with his elbow and, as a result, she could not eat solid foods for over three months.

Alicia shares that she knows that God had sent angels to protect her and that it just was not "her time to die." She says she felt a presence protecting her. Alicia slowly recovered from this incident, but the abuse did not stop. On several occasions, she says, Doug would tell her he was going to kill her, and would lie next to her, poking an ice pick in her back. She says she was terrified, and believed that at any moment he really would stab her. She also talks about severe sexual abuse. On many occasions Doug violently raped her, with their children present in the same small space that was their home. He forced her to stay in the tent for weeks at a time. The children were not allowed to attend school, and Alicia was not allowed to shower. Doug did not even allow her to go to the bathroom. He told her to go right were she was. Alicia says that her hair was matted and she was often soaked with her own urine. His method of controlling her was to stand at the tent opening with a gun, threatening to kill anyone who attempted to leave. Sometimes Doug allowed her to go in the store to buy food for the children, but Alicia says she would have to go in filthy, and smelling like urine. Even then, the same old routine was expected: Alicia had to walk in front of Doug, with her head covered and down.

Doug's spiritual abuse continued. Every word he spoke was about how evil his wife was, and how a woman should submit to her husband. He raped her and beat her almost to the point of death because she was not a "good" wife and was "evil." He was going to beat repentance into her. Alicia finally, miraculously escaped from Doug. She says that she saw the window of opportunity to escape, grabbed her children, and ran. As she was running, her oldest child again came to her defense, and lagged behind as he watched his father pull out his gun and aim it directly at her. Alicia says she remembers hearing her son screaming at his dad not to do it, as he was knocking the barrel of the gun down with his arm. She looked back but only for a second. Alicia left her oldest son behind with the man she called his father, the very man who had just tried to kill her.

Alicia reports that she hysterically ran into a convenience store and begged the people there to call for help. She reflects that the store owners "must have thought I was a madwoman, running into their store, hysterical, urine soaked, with matted hair and crying, children being dragged behind." Help came, as well as a safe place to stay, and clean clothing was provided. However, her oldest child was left behind. Alicia said she feared that Doug would either kill their son, or hold him hostage. Alicia went to the church that she and Doug had attended a few times, and asked for prayer. She says that she did not tell them the whole story because she was embarrassed. She told them only that her son was with his father and that it was not a safe place for him to be. The church held a prayer vigil, and Alicia says that within fifteen minutes her son was returned safely. Sadly, her son reported that Doug did indeed torment him for the three days he was alone with him. Doug kept him up the entire time "preaching" to him from the Bible. Alicia managed to take all her children to another battered women's shelter. When she entered the shelter this time, she was in much worse shape. She had head contusions from the numerous beatings. She had hand tremors. She had to wear diapers because of her inability to control her bladder and bowel functioning. She crawled out of bed in the mornings because her back pain was so excruciating that she could not walk. These were the effects of physical abuse. Alicia's children have told her that she slept with her eyes open. She also suffered severe anxiety attacks and nightmares.

Two years after completing the shelter program, Alicia has relocated and is living on her own. She has had no contact with Doug, but she is still suffering the effects of her abuse. Alicia made several suicide threats, which resulted in her being hospitalized twice. When asked why she wanted to die, her response was that she "just wanted peace." She still has trouble sleeping at night, and still suffers from anxiety attacks. She reports that she is on several psychiatric medications and they are helping. As for Alicia's spirituality, she reports that she knows she has been forgiven. It is tragic that Alicia still feels that she has sinned for leaving her husband and needs forgiveness. She reports that the biggest obstacle to her spirituality was feeling ashamed that she had "let the Father down" by breaking her marriage vows. Alicia still believes a woman should be submissive to a man. She has trouble talking to men, and cannot look them in the eyes. As for church, she says she does not attend much. Alicia shared that she is suspicious of church because Doug told her that churchgoers were often "wolves in sheep's clothing." Her faith in God, however, has miraculously withstood the ultimate test that Satan handed her. In the next chapter we will discuss demonic possession and its relation to domestic violence.

Chapter 11

Demonic Possession and Oppression

After reading Alicia's account of the abuse she suffered at the hands of her husband, and the obvious spiritual overtones of Doug's abuse, you may wonder what causes people to become so rigid and overbearing in their supposed Christianity. One of the most pervasive reasons why spiritual abuse occurs may be attributed to demonic activity. Several Scriptures give us insight into this spiritual aspect. One such Scripture is found in Mark 5, in which we read the account of Jesus' interaction with a demon-possessed man. This possessed man was evidently given a supernatural physical strength, was self-mutilating, and not in his "right mind" (Mark 5:3-5, Mark 5:15). The poor fellow was possessed by a legion of demons! When Jesus ordered the demons out of the man, they went into a herd of 2,000 pigs, which, in turn, ran into a lake and drowned themselves. This is evidence that demonic activity occurs with violence, and that demons have suicidal impulses, whether they possess men or animals. The account of this same story in Matthew reveals that the demon-possessed men "were so violent that no one could pass that way" (Matthew 8:28). Also, these Scriptures reveal that demon possession may include some form of mental derangement. People with mental disorders are not always demon possessed, but demon-possessed people almost always have some form of mental disorder. Demonic possession has symptoms of mental disorders, and also physical disorders.

In Matthew we read about a young boy who suffered from seizures that were attributed to demonic possession (Matthew 17:14-18). Luke describes this same boy as "foaming at the mouth," "screaming," and suffering from "convulsions" (Luke 9:39). We also read about a demon-possessed man who was mute, and was able to speak after the demon left him (Matthew 9:32-33), and a man who was blind due to demon possession (Matthew 12:22). Another account tells of a demon-possessed man who was yelling, and the demon actually threw the man down to the ground (Luke 4:33-35). All of these accounts reveal that there is always some mental and/or physical manifestation of the internal demonic activity of the possessed person. Again, that is not suggesting that blindness, or muteness, or seizures are due to demonic possession, but that one cannot be demon possessed and not show outward signs.

You may be left asking how one comes to be demon possessed. Unfortunately, none of the accounts previously mentioned give us any history on the possessed people, but we do have a few other accounts. One is found in the case of Judas. Judas was in the "inner circle" of Jesus' disciples and eventually betrayed Jesus, which led to Jesus' crucifixion. John 13:27 says that Satan entered Judas. Luke 22:3 says the same thing. On a side note, Judas committed suicide (Matthew 27:3-5; Acts 1:18). This indicated that Judas was very troubled at least, and possibly still possessed when he died. The account of Judas reveals that it was nothing Judas directly did that led to his possession. Satan just entered him. Only God knows why it was Judas, but we must understand that had Satan not entered one of the disciples, Jesus may never have died for us. Clearly, a higher purpose was intended. Whether God would have accomplished His purpose through other means is questionable, but the point is that Judas' Satanic possession was part of God's plan. That is not to say that possession is always part of God's plan or within God's will. An interesting distinction in the case of Judas' possession is that it was Satan himself who went into Judas. All other biblical accounts speak of demonic possession, not Satanic possession. Demons are the angels that went with Satan when he fell from heaven (Matthew 25:41). How does demonic possession happen?

Entire books have been written about demonic possession and spiritual warfare, but keeping in mind the purpose of this book, two distinct opportunities occur when people can become demon possessed. They both correlate strongly with the characteristics of batterers. The first, and most obvious, is the deep-rooted anger that batterers tend to possess. We know from Ephesians 4:26 and 27 that anger can be a potential "door" for Satan to walk through. The Scripture reads:

> In your anger do not sin: Do not let the sun go down while you are still angry, and do not give the devil a foothold.

When we allow ourselves to carry anger for any length of time, we may give the devil a foothold. We allow him to creep in, and once he is there, it is a battle to get him out. For the chronically angry person, it is a daily battle.

The second, and less obvious opportunity for demonic possession is related to the use of chemical substances. The use of drugs and alcohol by batterers is well documented. A study published by the National Institute of Justice, (Brookoff, 1997), revealed that 92 percent of abusers used drugs or alcohol the same day that they assaulted a family member. Indeed, substance abuse and domestic violence tend to go hand in hand. Although the Bible does not blatantly reveal anything about the use of drugs, God certainly speaks against drunkenness (Ephesians 5:18). Are being under the influence of chemicals, and being demon possessed entirely different?

Further study in God's word reveals that the use of drugs is the same as "witchcraft." Galatians 5:20 lists several things that we do in our sinful nature that cause our loss of inheritance to God's Kingdom. Among these, witchcraft is listed. As a side note, fits of rage are also on that list. Further study into the original language of the Bible shows us that the Greek word for "witchcraft" is *pharmakeia.* This word appears two other times, and is translated as sorceries in both Scriptures (Revelation 9:21 and 18:23). The actual Greek use of that word is also defined as "the use or the administering of drugs" and "poisoning." Hence, our English words "pharmacy" and "pharmaceuticals" are from the Greek root. The use of drugs is equated with witchcraft because the use of drugs opens a door to the soul, and God wants us to know this.

Any sin in our lives invites the wiles of Satan, whether through condemnation, further temptations, or any other Satanic strategy.

Quite simply, living in sin is contrary to living in the Spirit (Galations 5:16), and if you are not living in the Spirit, Satan may "drag you away" (James 1:14). The use of chemicals also opens the door by altering the thinking ability of the user. Remember that one of Satan's strategies is to attack our thoughts, and only when we are of a "sound mind" do we stand a chance of battling Satan. Ephesians 6:14 says that in order to stand our ground with Satan, we must put on "the belt of truth." It is nearly impossible to discern the truth when our brains are clouded with chemicals, so Satan gains a foothold when we open that door to him.

Opening a door to your soul does not always result in demon possession. There is a difference between being demon possessed and being oppressed by evil. The only other account besides that of Judas in which Satan "entered" an apparently godly man, was recorded in Matthew 16:23. Peter was speaking to the Lord, and His response to Peter was "Get behind me, Satan!" From this account, we gather that Peter was being oppressed by Satan at that moment, because the Bible makes no mention of Peter ever being demon possessed. Oppression occurs at various times in the lives of all Christians, and it comes in the various forms of Satanic strategies previously mentioned. Possession occurs when the person does not have the Holy Spirit indwelling. We know this from Jesus' teaching, as recorded in Matthew 12:43-45:

> When an evil spirit comes out of a man, it goes through arid places seeking rest and does not find it. Then it says, "I will return to the house I left." When it arrives, *it finds the house unoccupied, swept clean and put in order.* Then it goes and takes with it seven other spirits more wicked than itself, and they go and live there. And the final condition of that man is worse than the first (italics added).

The Scripture reveals several truths that pertain not only to demon possession, but domestic violence as well. First, it tells us that when our "house" is not being occupied by the Spirit, we are in grave danger of demon possession. It also reveals that even if a demon leaves a possessed person, it will come back with more demons. This Scripture speaks to the cycle of violence theory.

The cycle of violence is a common term used in psychology to describe the cycle that occurs within an abusive relationship. Once the abuse starts, a pattern is established. That pattern begins with a "tension phase," in which the abused partner senses the tension building in the relationship and the abuser. Something bad is about to happen. After a few times around this cycle, the abused partner is not just suspicious, but certain. Everyone in the home begins to tiptoe around the abuser. Sometimes the victim will become so filled with anxiety during this phase that she will almost beg the abuse to occur, just to get it over with. Then comes the "abuse phase." This can be a single battering, or a period of time with multiple types and incidences of abuse. Usually, the more times around the cycle, the longer the abuse phase becomes, to the point when it is the longest occurring phase of the cycle. Not only does the length of this phase increase, the level of abuse often increases. Then, the batterer begins to feel remorse or shame, and the "honeymoon phase" begins. During the honeymoon phase, the batterer showers his partner with love, affection, and gifts. He may even cry, and promise that he will never do it again. He may tell her how stupid he is, and that she is the best thing that ever happened to him. All of these statements and gestures reassure her that life is not really that bad, and after a period of time, she may completely discount the abuse phase. The honeymoon, however, does not last. The tension slowly starts building again, and the cycle continues, intensifying each time around. Eventually, the honeymoon phase is completely absent from the cycle, if the relationship endures that long.

Although we should not generalize, Jesus' teaching regarding the characteristics of demon possession seems similar to what we know about the characteristics of abusers caught in the cycle of violence. Although an abuser may feel a sense of remorse for his actions during the honeymoon phase, the Spirit is not necessarily within him at that point. The demon may leave for a time, and the abuser may have his house "swept clean and put in order," but he has not filled it with the Spirit, so the demon returns with seven more demons worse than itself, and they "find the house unoccupied." That is not to say that all abusers are demon possessed, but only that there are comparative similarities between what Jesus taught and the dynamics of the abusive marriage. We must be careful not to rely solely on the logic of similarities to determine if a person is demon possessed, but must rely more heavily on God's gift of discernment in our unique situations. We will discuss discernment in more depth in a later chapter.

Chapter 12

The Abusive Spouse:
Why Abuse Continues

Obviously, demonic possession is one answer to why abuse continues, but it is not the only answer because not all abusers are demon possessed. What about the abuser who has some evidence of the Spirit in his life? What about demonic oppression? What happens in the mind of the abuser from the "honeymoon phase" to the "tension phase" of the abuse cycle? Why does the abuser become abusive?

Abuse is about power and control. There may be several reasons why an abusive person seeks power and control in a relationship. One of these reasons is related to the abuser's own feelings of self-worth. Sometimes an abuser feels so inadequate or insecure that "forcing" his partner to stay guarantees she will never leave. That is obvious oppression by the enemy. It is Satan's subtle whisper that he is not worthy of being loved. Sometimes an abuser thinks that a woman is a second-class citizen, and as his wife, she becomes his property. This type of abuser will use the Ephesians and Colossians Scriptures to justify his controlling behavior. Again, this is Satan's subtle twisting of the Scripture to thwart the true will of God. Sometimes an abuser just wants things done his way, and has little patience for or acceptance of alternatives. This may be a hardening of the heart, or a situation of self-will run awry. Again, this is based on a lie from Satan that we know what is best in our own lives, and are in complete control. Sometimes an abuser has deep-seated anger and resentment that is displaced on his partner. This type of abuser may feel as if he is a victim. Life has treated him unfairly. This is yet another lie from Satan.

Some of these abusers are "overcontrolled." They allow the oppression to fester, until they finally weaken unto it, and then they explode with a fierceness that can be very dangerous. Some of these abusers have no control at all, and lash out at the first sign of oppression. Some abusers possess all of these traits, and some possess a few, or only one. The oppression almost always comes in the area of "sensitivity" that is unique to the abuser. However, the effectiveness of Satan's strategy is not in the individual weakness of the abuser. It is in the disabling of the abuser's ability to fight against the oppression.

Psychologists refer to "defense mechanisms" as the tools we use to fend off attacks to the "self" or "ego." God calls it "will." This theory, from a spiritual perspective, is another Satanic lie. In God we have no "self," so we really need no protection. Our protection comes from God and God alone, and is not based on our own identity, but on our *identity in God*. We need protection only for our souls, not our will, and only God can provide that for us. Satan would like us to continue to protect our free will ("self," "ego") because then we may continue to rebel against God. In the arena of domestic violence, "defense mechanisms" run deep.

Psychologists have identified several defense mechanisms, but a few are more common among batterers.

- *Minimization.* This defense occurs when the abuser minimizes his abuse. "Well, I never hit her." "I didn't even leave a bruise." "I only threatened her. I didn't really follow through."
- *Denial.* The abuser completely denies his own abusive behavior, as if it never happened. This type of defense prevents the abuser from ever coming to repentance because he does not even admit to having a problem.
- *Blaming.* By blaming his partner for his own abusive behaviors, he protects himself from taking responsibility for the abuse.
- *Rationalization.* This behavior often occurs in Christian homes when the abuser uses Scripture to rationalize that his abusiveness is actually God's will.

All of these defense mechanisms have one thing in common. They hinder the ability of the Spirit to bring the abuser to repentance, and they allow Satan to continue his oppressing forces. In fact, they are a manifestation of Satan's "core" sin. Remember our discussion on why Satan fell from heaven? Pride. The abuser's pride is the rudimentary force behind his defense mechanisms. This pride can also be linked to Adam's lack of accountability in the Garden of Eden. It is evidence of Satan's influence upon us. Not only the abusive person in the relationship experiences demonic oppression or uses defense mechanisms. The abused also does.

Chapter 13

The Abused Spouse: Spiritual Justifications for Abuse

We cannot discuss domestic violence without addressing the family perspective, especially when we consider it in a spiritual light. The husband and wife become "one," and in that sense, the one affects the other. That does not imply that the abused spouse is to blame for the abuse. Accountability must be accepted by the abusing spouse. On the other hand, abuse continues because it is allowed to continue. Remember, women tend to stay in abusive relationships because they fear severe retaliation if they attempt to leave. They also tend to stay because of the children, or for economic and/or emotional reasons. For the Christian woman the reasons are more strongly tied to her beliefs, rooted in her spirituality, and fundamental to her relationship with God. Often, these reasons are weapons used by Satan in his warfare strategy, and he uses them either directly or through the church. Satanic strategies will be exposed in this chapter.

Many Christian women who are or have been in an abusive relationship stayed because they accepted the abuse as "the cross they must carry." This belief comes from the teaching of Jesus, as recorded in Matthew 10:38, Matthew 16:24, Mark 8:34, Luke 9:23, and Luke 14:27. Luke 14:27 reads:

> And anyone who does not carry his cross and follow me cannot be my disciple.

The other Scriptures listed are worded similarly. This is a very important spiritual principle Jesus was teaching, yet it is often misunderstood and mistaught, particularly in the context we are discussing. Think about what carrying a cross literally means. It ultimately means death. Anyone who is carrying a cross is probably carrying it to the place where it will be anchored to the ground, and the carrier will be nailed to it until death. Jesus is teaching us to be willing to carry the burden or pain of death. Other Scriptures record Jesus' teaching on this. For example, in Matthew 16:24-25 it is written:

> If anyone would come after me, he must deny himself and take up his cross and follow me. For whoever wants to save his life will lose it, but whoever loses his life for me will find it.

What does this mean? Jesus did not mean literal death, although sometimes that is the price of following Jesus. Most of the disciples were persecuted until death because of their faith. In this passage Jesus implied death to the self. He says "you must deny yourself if you want to follow me." That is the cross He says we must carry. Imagine walking up a hill carrying a heavy cross on your back, knowing you are carrying that cross to your own death. What does that image mean to you? It probably represents a deep commitment to God that you are turning over your own will and surrendering to His. That is not easy for some of us to do, and Jesus knew that. Surrendering to God's will is not the same as suffering in the name of martyrdom. Although God does call certain individuals to martyrdom, carrying our cross does not usually mean submitting to every ill circumstance in life. It certainly does not mean that God's will is for us to be abused as the "cross" we must bear.

Other Scriptures used to erroneously validate staying in an abusive relationship are ones that refer to the sufferings of being a Christian. Some of these are found in 1 Peter 3:13+. Peter writes: "But even if you should suffer for doing right, you are blessed" (1 Peter 3:14). What is right? He also writes: "It is better, if it is God's will, to suffer for doing good than for doing evil" (1 Peter 3:17). What is God's will? And finally, Peter writes: "Therefore, since Christ suffered in his body, arm yourselves also with the same attitude—" (1 Peter 4:1). The attitude *of* suffering? Not exactly. Peter was referring to the attitude *toward* suffering, which the Lord adopted, and suffering because of ultimate submission to God's will. Suffering on the cross to be obedient to His father's will is the attitude that Peter refers to. Again, the theme is dying to self, and the inspired Word of God acknowledges that dying to self often requires some amount of suffering. God's will in and of itself does not mean we must suffer. Jesus demonstrated the ultimate act of submission, and suffering through physical pain accompanied His submission. That obviously is no ordinary act. In fact, it is so unordinary that God reserved it for His Son. We, as Christians, do not have to suffer physical pain in order to be in submission to God's will. However, we must be *willing* to suffer if that is what God calls us to do.

The catch here is knowing what God calls us to do, knowing what His will is, both expressed and implied. We will address this in more depth in the next section but, for now, understand that these Scriptures of Peter's, and others like them, are not saying that Christians *must* suffer, but only that Christians must be in submission to God, *even if that means suffering.* When you understand the Scriptures from that perspective, it almost seems preposterous to attempt to apply this spiritual principle to a situation of family abuse, unless one truly believes that it is God's will to remain in an abusive relationship.

Sadly, many people do believe that it is God's will for an abused wife to remain in the abusive relationship. Scriptures that refute this belief will be discussed in the next section, but let us first explore this idea from a humanistic point of view. A popular story was told to me by a Pastor when I was seeking marriage counseling. It is also told in a few books, all intended to illustrate the above spiritual principle.

A man was in the bar one night. He made a bet with two of his friends that if they all went to his house he could make his wife get up out of bed and fix something to eat for all of them. Not only that, but she would get up and do it without complaint. Who would refuse a bet like this? So the three of them, drunk, stagger into the guy's house sometime past 2 a.m. He goes into the bedroom, and out comes his wife with a smile. She goes into the kitchen, still with a smile, and cooks them all dinner. The two friends could not believe it! They paid the bet, and then asked the wife how she could seem so pleasant under the circumstances. The wife revealed that she is a Christian, and that the husband not being a Christian made her want to be more of an example of Jesus to him. The story ends with the husband becoming so convicted by his wife's attitude that he also becomes a Christian.

That is a nice story to illustrate an important spiritual principle, but if taken literally that type of circumstance is not only abusive, the wife's behavior is an impossible standard to live up to day after day. Granted, once or twice may be tolerable, but anyone who has lived with an alcoholic knows that alcoholic behaviors never get better on their own. If the husband thought he could do that to his wife and still be allowed in the house, then it probably was not the first time he had done it. In fact, he bet on it. He already knew that he could do that to his wife and get away with it. Why would he suddenly, based on this one incident, become convicted when he obviously already knew her pattern of "godly" behavior? Nothing had worked before, but now he suddenly becomes convicted? Conviction is from God and God alone. The fine point here is that sometimes our godly behavior in the face of adversity *is* a testimony, but sometimes it is just an opportunity for Satan to laugh at us. Knowing the difference between when our submission will be a testimony, and when it will be taken for granted requires discernment. Also, knowing when something is God's will requires discernment. Often, though, it is so obvious that it requires only honesty with God and ourselves.

Another common reason Christian women stay in an abusive relationship is related to forgiveness. Obviously, the wife in the above story either did not feel at all hurt by her husband's behavior, or she did, but forgave him. More likely, she forgave him. Forgiveness is the main ingredient in our decisions to personally accept God's brand of salvation, and it is also a fundamental Christian principle that is well illustrated throughout the Bible. When Peter asked Jesus how many times he should forgive someone who sins against him, Jesus replied: "I tell you, not seven times, but seventy-seven times" (Matthew 18:22). This Scripture seems to imply that we should always forgive. Luke's account of this teaching gives a slightly different picture. It is recorded in Luke 17:3 and 4:

> If your brother sins, *rebuke him, and if he repents, forgive him.* If he sins against you seven times in a day, and seven times comes back to you and says, "I repent," forgive him (italics added).

If he repents is the key here.

Luke also tells us the beautiful story of a sinful woman who came to Jesus and worshipped at His feet. Because of her love for Jesus, He said that her many sins had been forgiven (Luke 7:36-50). We see in this story a true heart of repentance. What exactly is repentance? The Greek word used in the above Scripture is *metanoeo* and it means: "to change one's mind, or, to change one's mind for better, heartily to amend with abhorrence of one's past sins." To abhor means to hate, or dislike. Therefore, repentance means we come to hate our own sin so much that we change our mind about it. It is a done deal and not easily forsaken. Paul wrote to the Corinthians that "Godly sorrow brings about repentance that leads to salvation and leaves no regret, but worldly sorrow brings death" (2 Corinthians 7:10). True godly sorrow saves us from our own sin. We stop committing that same sin that we are repentant about. To illustrate this principle, consider the man who sits on death row for murder, who is in tears over his crime. True repentance means the man recognized his sinfulness and came to a place of sorrow over it; worldly repentance means the man was sorry for murdering because he is on death row. The same holds true for the batterer. Is he truly experiencing repentance, or is he sorry that he may lose his family?

Another distinction must be made regarding forgiveness. Much confusion comes from misunderstanding the difference between forgiveness and acceptance. Satan capitalizes on the confusion. Unforgiveness leads to bitterness and resentment. It is harmful to our souls, and hinders our walk with God. We need to forgive every sin against us (Mark 11:25). However, that does not mean we accept the sin. Luke 17:3 and 4 tell us to forgive as many times as the person who sinned against us repents. However, these verses do not imply that the forgiveness is for the same sin. Seven different sins, seven acts of forgiveness. When the same sin is committed over and over, true repentance may not have occurred. Satan would like the abused spouse to continue to accept the oppression in the home. His foothold grows stronger each time she accepts. When she does not accept, his condemnation of her "unforgiveness" causes her to allow the abuse one more time. She may even start to believe that the abuse is her fault because she has not been forgiving enough.

Sadly, this may even be perpetuated by church doctrine. The doctrine of forgiveness is often based on the "law of nonresistance," found in Matthew 5:38-39:

> You have heard that it was said, "Eye for eye, and tooth for tooth." But I tell you, Do not resist an evil person. If someone strikes you on the right cheek, turn to him the other also.

This verse may cause a battered woman to think that if she is godly enough, she would just take the abuse and turn her other cheek. That is not exactly what these verses mean. The context of Jesus' teaching is not that you allow yourself to be abused, but that you should not repay evil with evil. In other words, do not strike back out of spite. Self-defense and intentional harm are entirely different, and although we may have a difficult time discerning between the two in a court of law, God already knows our heart's intention, and if we are honest with ourselves, so do we.

Another common doctrine that may be used to oppress the abused spouse relates to judgment. She may believe that she has no right to "judge" her husband, and without that judgment, she is immobilized to take action in the relationship. Several verses speak against judgment, such as Luke 6:37: "Do not judge, and you will not be judged." Likewise, it is written in Matthew 7:1-2:

> Do not judge, or you too will be judged. For in the same way you judge others, you will be judged, and with the measure you use, it will be measured to you.

Jesus almost seems harsh in these and the next three verses. He has reason to be harsh. Although He is saying that we should not judge others, He is speaking about a defense mechanism that psychologists call "projection." When we see our own "character flaws" in other people, but not in ourselves, we are projecting. We pass judgment on others for committing the same sins we ourselves commit. Jesus is clearly saying not to do that. Clean our own side of the street, so to speak, before we point out the garbage on the other side of the street. This teaching may be used to imply that we should not look on the other side of the street at all, but looking and passing judgment about what we see are two different issues.

Think about our legal system. What does a judge do? A judge may make two decisions. The first is determining the person's guilt. That is often obvious if enough evidence is presented. The most important decision, however, is determining the fate of the person. The judge decides the punishment. In the spiritual realm, only God can sit in that seat. It is not for us to say if a person will go to heaven or hell. Only God knows the state of our hearts and our motives, so ultimately He makes judgment about guilt. However, God clearly instructs us to make some judgment, because He tells us in 1 Corinthians 2:15:

> The spiritual man makes judgments about all things, but he himself is not subject to any man's judgment.

If God did not want us to make some judgments, He never would have given the gift of discernment. In this sense, it is not our flesh that makes the judgment, but the Spirit of God within us. Within this arena, our judgments are righteous. Satan would once again like to condemn us for passing judgment, because he knows that we may discern between spirits, and uncover the true oppression within the home.

Another reason the abused spouse may stay in the relationship is related to love and the heart. Love is powerful. The *agape* love of God is a healing force. Indeed, the Scriptures tell us that God is love (1 John 4:8). However, as we most often perceive it, love is an emotion. God created woman to be more emotional than man. This is where confusion may enter. Because God is love, and an abused spouse may feel an intense love for her husband, she may believe that the love she feels is "from God." This may justify her staying in the relationship, even when there is no evidence of repentance in her husband's life. God warns us not to trust our hearts because "the heart is deceitful above all things and beyond cure" (Jeremiah 17:9). Woman's greatest strengths are her abilities to show compassion, to nurture, and to love, but these are also her weakest points in terms of warfare strategy. Satan will use this information to accuse abused women, who often think that the situation will remedy itself if they only learn to "love" more. This belief may be perpetuated by Scriptures such as 1 Peter 4:8: "Above all, love each other deeply, because love covers over a multitude of sins." The love referred to here is the *agape* love of God; however, it is actually translated as "charity" in the King James Bible. This verse may cause an abused spouse to think that her love is strong enough to sustain the relationship. She is trying to "love" enough for both of them. The problem is that she is taking over his responsibility. She is fervently trying to cover his sin for him, which leads us to the primary reason she may stay in the relationship.

The abused spouse often perceives that she is to blame for the abuse. "If only I was more submissive, more forgiving, more compassionate, more loving, he would change." In a sense, she is trying to emulate the personhood of Christ, which is what we, as Christians, are supposed to do. We continually allow God to change us to be more like Him. 1 John 2:6 reads: "Whoever claims to live in Him must walk as Jesus did." In all situations and relationships, we must ask ourselves, "What would Jesus do?" However, an intimate knowledge of the personhood of Him is required first. This is where misunderstanding takes hold. In the abusive relationship, the abused partner may be adopting the characteristics of Jesus, but she may take on the responsibility for "saving" the abusive spouse. This is a "Savior Complex." Desiring to be like Jesus is not against what God wants us to do, but doing it because we think we can "save" or change someone else through our own actions is. There is only one Savior, and only He can save souls. God will use our actions as testimony to others, but this is not His only means. Testimony means nothing to a heart that is hardened toward God. If an abuser is not held accountable for the abuse, repentance may never occur. In other words, God works more readily in the heart that is broken, and constantly "shielding" the abuser from getting to that point is preventing God from being able to work in the heart.

These doctrines tend to lead a woman living in domestic violence to self-blame. "If only I had been more forgiving, more submissive, more tolerant." "If only I could hang in there a little longer and pray a little more." Or even worse, "if only I had more faith that God would change him." These are the lies of the enemy and, sadly, are perpetuated through misunderstanding of Scripture. This is why God's word is so "inconsistent," as Bible skeptics would say. It is not that God's word is inconsistent, as much as it balanced. For many Scriptures, there are opposite Scriptures. Understanding both perspectives provides balance and, hopefully, the wisdom to apply it.

The final reason why women stay in abusive relationships, and one which also will be addressed more specifically later, centers around divorce. Most Christians shudder at the word and the seriousness of the thought. Divorce is often taught within the church to be a taboo and horrible sin, so a woman may think that she has no choices. Indeed, the church often gives her no other choice. Biblical choices are available. We will examine these in the next section.

SECTION IV:
GOD'S PLANS AND INSTRUCTIONS
FOR A TROUBLED RELATIONSHIP

Chapter 14

Spiritual Armor

Both demonic oppression and possession require a certain level of personal accountability. Both the abused and the abuser must take responsibility for their part in the cycle of violence within the relationship. Ultimately God fights the spiritual battles we face, but we must be "team players" or the battle is futile. We must not slump down in defeated surrender, but must stand tall and unafraid. 2 Timothy 1:7 tells us, "God did not give us a spirit of timidity, but a spirit of power, of love and of self-discipline." These are all very strong characteristics that God gives us, and He expects us to use them.

However, we cannot fight the battle and expect to win just because we stand tall. The most important truth to remember when caught in the midst of spiritual warfare is that God does the rescuing. It is written in 2 Timothy 4:18: "The Lord will rescue me from every evil attack and will bring me safely to his heavenly kingdom." The Lord will. Surely if we could rescue ourselves, God would have no place in our lives. Why does God rescue us? Luke 1:74 tells us that He does because He wants us to be able to serve Him without fear. Servanthood. Because we serve Him, He rescues us (Psalm 91:14). What happens when we do not serve Him?

Jesus said, as recorded in Luke 12:4-5, "I tell you, my friends, do not be afraid of those who kill the body and after that can do no more. But I will show you whom you should fear: Fear him who, after the killing of the body, has power to throw you into hell." Jesus immediately explains the consequences of not serving him (Luke12:8+). In order to have a chance against Satan, we must have God on our side, and we must do our part within the army of God.

Before we go into the specifics of spiritual armor, let us examine Jesus' instruction that we should not fear "those who kill the body but can do no more" (Luke 12:4). From this Scripture we may adopt the doctrine that we should not ever fear those who may hurt us. Fear is a legitimate human emotion that God created within us to serve a purpose. It warns us of danger, and can sometimes be a prompting by the Holy Spirit to take action to protect ourselves. Proverbs 29:25 says, "Fear of man will prove to be a snare, but whoever trusts in the Lord is kept safe." These Scriptures show us that we should not be afraid of dying, but should be afraid of going to hell.

Does that mean we should not even attempt to avoid death? These Scriptures may cause an abused woman to remain in a potentially lethal relationship because she assumes that if she is afraid of her husband, she is not living up to God's standards. She may consciously deny her fear in order to live a life she feels is more godly. In turn, for an abuser, these Scriptures may be used as tools to attack her faith by trivializing her fear of him by telling her that it is not biblical to be afraid of him. That doctrine would purport that standing in front of an oncoming train is acceptable because we should not fear death, and God will rescue us. It would also tell us that if someone breaks into our home while we are sleeping, and attempts to stab our children, we should not fight back or be afraid. Is that what God meant when He gave us these Scriptures?

Fear of physical harm is entirely different from fear of God or Satan. This distinction is most clear in 2 Corinthians 10:4:

The weapons we fight with are not weapons of the world.

In other words, our battle is not in the physical realm, but in the spiritual. Paul reiterates this in Ephesians 6:12:

For our struggle is not against flesh and blood, but against the rulers, against the authorities, against the powers of this dark world and against the spiritual forces of evil in the heavenly realms.

These verses tell us that although a battle may seem physical, as Christians, our true struggles come from spiritual battles. Spiritual battles are not always manifested in the physical realm, but sometimes they are. When they are physical we should not just allow ourselves to be physically overcome by our enemies. We should recognize that the battle is spiritual, and requires spiritual armor. A battered woman may have no physical armor to protect her at all, but she is responsible to put on spiritual armor. Likewise, although the abusive spouse may be under demonic possession or oppression, he is still responsible to fight off the spiritual attack upon himself by putting on the same spiritual armor.

Following the above Ephesians Scripture, Paul explains what the spiritual armor is (Ephesians 6:14-18). First, he says, put on the "belt of truth buckled around your waist." This first piece of armor has implications for further discussion, and we will come back to it later. The second piece of armor Paul lists is the "breastplate of righteousness." Righteousness is obtained through accepting Jesus as our Savior (2 Corinthians 5:21). Because Jesus is righteous and we as Christians abide in Him, we take on His attribute of righteousness. We did not earn it on our own. We are not righteous on our own (Romans 3:10). Jesus is righteous and through our faith in Him, we are also made righteous (Romans 3:22). We are to place this "breastplate" of righteousness over us. A breastplate protects the breast, one of the most vital areas of our bodies. Our breasts enclose our hearts, and all other vital organs. God instructs us to guard our hearts. "Above all else, guard your heart, for it is the wellspring of life" (Proverbs 4:23). We guard our hearts by putting Jesus' righteousness over us.

Paul also tells us to have our "feet fitted with the readiness that comes from the gospel of peace" (Ephesians 5:15). A soldier's armor in biblical times included brass-type shoes that prevented him from being stuck in the foot with sharp sticks and gall traps which were laid in the path of marching armies. Once stuck, the soldier could no longer march forward. Paul is instructing us to place protection on our feet because if we do not, we may be rendered immobile. Also, Paul is suggesting that we must be ready to move forward. We get ready through the gospel.

Paul next instructs us to put on the shield of faith. Paul further tells us that this shield should be used to "extinguish all the flaming arrows of the evil one" (Ephesians 5:16). Faith is the one piece of armor that makes all the others useful. We must have faith for all of the other pieces to work effectively. Without faith we have no truth, no righteousness, no readiness. Faith is not just picked up off the ground. Hebrews 12:2 says, "Let us fix our eyes on Jesus, the author and perfecter of our faith—." Jesus is the author of our faith. He created it. He molds it.

The next piece of armor listed is the helmet of salvation. A helmet protects the head, and the head houses the brain. Remember that one of Satan's strategies is to meddle with our thoughts. We protect ourselves by putting on the helmet of salvation. Refer to 2 Corinthians 10:5. Paul says that "we demolish arguments and every pretension that sets itself up against the knowledge of God, and we take captive every thought to make it obedient to Christ." We do that by putting on the helmet of salvation.

The final piece of armor Paul lists is actually a weapon. It is the "sword of the Spirit, which is the word of God" (Ephesians 5:17). The sword of God is His word, and it is the only weapon we have that is used in both defense and offense.

Before we further discuss the "belt of truth," we need to make some general observations about God's metaphor for spiritual armor. First, notice that none of the pieces of our armor are manmade. Because they exist in a spiritual realm, they belong to God. He created them, and He gives them to us. Also notice, however, that we must put them on ourselves. They are useless unless we put them on, and God will not do that for us. Note that if we do not put on every piece of armor, if we exclude even one, we leave ourselves vulnerable to attack. The enemy is more likely to prevail where we are weakest. Finally, notice that there is no armor for our backside. That tells us to never turn our backs on Satan. Perhaps that is why Paul said "stand your ground" (Ephesians 6:13). Does that mean that an abused spouse should never "turn her back" on her abuser? No. Remember, this Scripture is in the context of the spiritual realm, and not the literal realm of the flesh. The point is that we do not surrender in the battle by turning our back on Satan.

Now, let us return to the "belt of truth." What does God mean by "truth"? The Greek word that is used in this Scripture has several meanings. The most fitting definitions according to *Strong's Concordance* are: (1) "what is true in things appertaining to God and the duties of man, moral and religious truth"; (2) "the true notions of God which are open to human reason without his supernatural intervention"; and (3) "that candour of mind which is free from affection, pretence, simulation, falsehood, deceit." In other words, we have truth with a capital "T," and the inner truth that comes from repentance. The Truth of God is an essential element in spiritual battle. We must be able to discern between the Truth of God and the lie of the enemy. What is a belt used for? It keeps everything in place. What happens when our pants are too big and we do not have a belt or we wear a robe without the belt around it? Parts of us become exposed and we become embarrassed or ashamed. The belt of truth is not meant to keep the lie within, so we are not embarrassed and ashamed, but rather the belt of truth exposes the lie. Truth exposes lies, as light exposes darkness. When we use the belt of truth to radiate all darkness within and around us, we send the enemy away. We may expose ourselves, but we are not ashamed. The enemy condemns. In more practical terms, we cannot wear the belt of truth if we are full of lies. We first must confess our sins. Through confession we illuminate the darkness within ourselves, and the bind that Satan once had on us is broken (Ephesians 5:11). Confession and repentance are essential aspects of truth. They are also essential elements for healing in an abusive relationship, as we will see in the next chapter.

Chapter 15

The Accountability of the Abuser: Repentance and Forgiveness

Before healing can begin in a marriage the source of the wound must be removed. If the source is marital infidelity, the infidelity must stop and must be replaced with faithfulness. If it is drug addiction, the drug must be surrendered, and replaced with God addiction. If it is domestic violence, the violence must stop and be replaced with healthier conflict resolutions. However, the process of getting from one side of the fence to the other is not a simple matter of will. If it was that simple, we would not need God at all. Indeed, most abusers do not want to hurt the people they love. Some of them are trying desperately to keep their spouse from leaving, yet their rational thought process says that if they continue to abuse, their spouse will leave. Then they abuse anyway. It does not make sense. It is similar to being told that if you touch the stove you will get burned, but you touch it anyway. What would make a person do that? In the psychological realm, we might call it addiction. It is so powerful that it is resistant to logic and rationality. Even the fear of the consequence cannot stop an addiction in full form. However, God does not call it addiction. He calls it sin. Sin always begins with a small step in the wrong direction. We are slowly desensitized to the consequences when we see that they are not that bad. With this desensitization comes a gradual increase in the sin, or addictive behavior. Once at full form, it has control of us, and we have lost control of it ("Jesus replied, 'I tell you the truth, everyone who sins is a slave to sin'" John 8:34). Domestic violence can be an addictive pattern of behavior. This is not always the case. Some individuals may be abusive because they truly believe they are "right" in their abusiveness. Perhaps they have been taught that as children. Once an abuser learns, through the criminal justice system, friends, family, the spouse, or church, that the abusive behavior is wrong, we would expect it to stop, yet it does not. We see evidence of this in the "cycle of violence" discussed in Chapter 11. The abusive spouse, during the "honeymoon" phase of the cycle, seems remorseful. He can see the damage his abusiveness is doing to his partner, to their relationship, and to the children. This cycle, however, is still in motion; the tension mounts until the abuse occurs again. Like a perpetual downward spiral, it does not stop. When it does not stop, or the abuser cannot stop it, there is indication that it is an addictive behavior. What does God say about addictive, or sinful behaviors?

When we are caught up in sin, our only hope of being saved from it is repentance. In addition to being saved from our sin, we are saved from hell. If we do not repent, we will suffer eternal life alone ("But unless you repent, you too will all perish" Luke 13:3). Remember Chapter 13 on the spiritual justifications for abuse. We discussed godly sorrow versus worldly sorrow in terms of repentance. The difference was illustrated through the example of the man on death row for murder. The cycle of violence is evidence that worldly sorrow, not godly sorrow, occurs in the abusive relationship. "Godly sorrow brings repentance that leads to salvation and leaves no regret . . ." (2 Corinthians 7:10). Repentance literally means that the sin is stopped. The real key here is that the sorrow is godly and not of man. It can come only from God, and thus requires God's divine intervention. We cannot achieve godly sorrow on our own fleshly accords. However, the lack of godly sorrow in one's life is not an indication that it is God's will for the sin to continue. God allows us every opportunity to repent, and when we do not, He "gives us over to a depraved mind" (Romans 1:28). He casts us away as unfit, and allows us to suffer the consequences of our own sin. He will only warn us so many times. How does God warn us?

God warns us through others, both believers and unbelievers, through prayer time with Him, and through Scripture. Several

Scriptures warn against abusiveness, or speak about it in terms of our sinfulness. Here are a few of them:

> The good man brings good things out of the good stored up in his heart, and the evil man brings evil things out of the evil stored in his heart. For out of the overflow of his heart his mouth speaks (Luke 6:45).

> . . . But I tell you that men will have to give account on the day of judgment for every careless word they have spoken (Matthew 12:36).

> Everyone should be quick to listen, slow to speak and slow to become angry, for man's anger does not bring about the righteous life that God desires (James 1:19).

> In your anger do not sin (Ephesians 4:26).

> Get rid of all bitterness, rage and anger . . . (Ephesians 4:31).

> A fool gives full vent to his anger, but a wise man keeps himself under control (Proverbs 29:11).

The same theme is written throughout God's word, pertaining to anger, our loose tongues, and physical and sexual abuse. It is definitely not in God's character to abuse. Paul wrote that we need to "be imitators of God" (Ephesians 5:1), and, as discussed in the first few chapters, God holds the man more accountable for this imitation as a leader within the marital relationship. Woman imitates the church, and man imitates Christ (Ephesians 5:22-26). But, what does it mean, other than sacrificing ourselves, to imitate God? In relation to domestic violence, several Scriptures describe God as "slow to anger and abounding in love" (Exodus 34:6, Numbers 14:18, Nehemiah 9:17, Psalms 86:15, Psalms 103:8, Jonah 4:2). Imitators of God should be slow to anger and abounding in love. Anything less is outside of His will, and detrimental to the marital relationship.

How do you determine if you are an abuser, and if you do, then what? God says to "examine yourselves to see whether you are in the faith; test yourselves" (2 Corinthians 13:5). You must first examine yourself in light of God's word. "But everything exposed by the light becomes visible, for it is light that makes everything visible" (Ephesians 5:13). Ask yourself if your behavior lines up with Scripture? James 1:22-24 warns: "Do not merely listen to the word, and so deceive yourselves. Do what it says. Anyone who listens to the word but does not do what it says is like a man who looks at his face in a mirror and, after looking at himself, goes away and immediately forgets what he looks like."

Have you ever examined yourself, found your short-comings, but then forgot how serious those faults were? When we forget who we really are, we forget how much we need a Savior, and we quickly fall back into self-reliance as a mode of coping with our lives. In the midst of addiction, self-reliance spirals us farther into the depths of sin. God created us to be addicts, but not addicts of the sinful nature of the world and its various trappings. Rather, God created us to be addicted to Him. We need God. Sometimes the only way we can remember that we need Him is by holding up that mirror in front of our faces daily. We must be in the word.

Another form of mirroring occurs through the Holy Spirit working among the fellowship of believers. James 5:16 tells us to "confess our sins to each other and pray for each other so that you may be healed." When we share our sins with other believers, a healing occurs. First, our darkness is exposed. Second, we become more accountable to fellow believers. Third, God hears specific and individualized prayer from other believers. James 5:16 also tells us that "the prayer of a righteous man is powerful and effective." Through all of these actions we are healed from our sin.

If you are abusive to your spouse, children, or parents, you may be thinking, "Well, I regularly confess my sin to my family. I always tell them how wrong I am and how sorry I am." That confession may be encouraging, but it is not enough to stop the abusive behavior.

Perhaps you counsel or mentor a couple who is in an abusive marriage. Search the Scriptures to understand the nature of domestic violence. Discern the presence of abuse in the relationship. A couple may be present for counseling, but the wife is afraid to discuss the true nature of the husband's behavior because of the repercussions when she returns home, and because she does not want to make him look bad in front of other people.

Domestic violence is an addiction that is interwoven into the dynamics of familial relationships. The problem may begin with one person in the family, but it quickly becomes a family problem. Again, God created man and woman to function as "one." If only one is confessing, in the case of domestic violence, no real accountability is taking place. This is in part due to the order God established, because man is not accountable to woman, but to God. It is also in part due to the "hidden" nature of family abuse. The secret stays within the family, and the entire family remains in darkness. This is perpetuated by the abuser's belief that his wife truly "loves" him because she continues to forgive. Remember that "[She] who covers over an offense promotes love, but whoever repeats the matter separates close friends" (Proverbs 17:9). The abuser needs to understand that his unrepentance is tearing the family down.

To truly expose the sin to light, the husband needs to confess his sin to another man within the church body. Most often an abusive man has difficulty doing this because of his pride. How comfortable he feels confessing his sins depends largely on his salvation. If the abusive spouse is not saved, there may be little hope outside of God that repentance will occur. However, if the abuser confesses his sins to a male church member who can guide him, he may be led to repentance, which leads to accepting salvation. Remember that God says that "there will be more rejoicing in heaven over one sinner who repents than over ninety-nine righteous persons who do not need to repent" (Luke 15:7). What if his pride is too strong, and he refuses to repent? That question will be answered in the next chapter.

Chapter 16

The Accountability of the Abused: Accepting Leadership

Just as the abuser must accept responsibility for the abuse, so also must the abused. Although the abuser is the primary person responsible for stopping the abuse, especially if the abuser is the husband or the spiritual leader, nothing can make him accept that responsibility. His lack of spiritual leadership, however, does not mean the entire family must go astray with him. Unfortunately, the family often does go astray, but not for the reasons we might initially think. One of the reasons we might assume is cobattering. Indeed, research indicates that females who are assaultive to their partners are most often in a situation of self-defense, or a long-standing pattern exists in the relationship of male-initiated domestic violence (Barnett, Keyson, and Thelen, 1992). People tend to adopt the behaviors and styles of resolving conflict that surround them. Desensitization occurs after time, as the husband's abuse becomes worse, and the wife may also begin to behave abusively. That is no excuse. If an abused wife becomes abusive, she is just as accountable for her abusiveness as is her husband. This is what Jesus was referring to when he said, "You have heard that it was said, 'Eye for eye, and tooth for tooth.' But I tell you, do not resist an evil person. If someone strikes you on the right cheek, turn to him the other also" (Matthew 5:38-39). (Also see Romans 12:17-21 for additional text on this spiritual principle.) God never approves of abuse, even when it is in response to another's abuse. Self-defense in a life-threatening situation is not the issue here. We are talking about a revengeful heart. However, this type of reaction is probably the least common for the abused Christian wife.

The spiritual problems in Christian families in the throes of domestic violence are related to the biblical misinterpretations we discussed in Chapter 13. Many of these misinterpretations develop into a common pattern of thinking and behaving for the abused spouse. The secular term for this is the "battered woman's syndrome." Another very popular term for a pattern of behavior with very similar characteristics is "codependency." God speaks about these behaviors. Very simply, He calls them sins. Just as the abuser, the abused spouse must be held accountable for her sin. Secular theories about codependency and the battered woman's syndrome suggest that the conditions are caused by abuse. We also must recognize an accountability factor for the victim of abuse. Accountability does not suggest blame. It only suggests that we are responsible for our own actions. Accountability does not mean that the victim of domestic violence is responsible for the abuse, but she is responsible to make appropriate decisions in her life. Most counselors would agree on this. However, distinctions exist between worldly counsel and biblical counsel regarding what an abused and/or codependent woman should be accountable for.

Secular counselors may urge codependents to rightfully take the focus of their life off of their partner, but erroneously urge them to place it on "self." "Think of yourself first." "Build your self-esteem." This Satanic strategy promotes the notion that we are in control of our lives, that we are responsible for our own healing, that we must save ourselves from our codependency, and that all we need to do is learn to "detach." God certainly would not argue against the idea that we detach ourselves from harmful relationships.

However, remember that God's perfect design for marriage calls for attachment even to the point of what psychologists call "enmeshment." In the realm of secular psychology, enmeshment is negative and unhealthy. Enmeshment occurs when each partner becomes so involved with the other that both lose their individual identities. The so-called boundaries of self become blurred in an enmeshed relationship. This is the crux of codependency. In some ways the idea of codependency is what God defines as His plan for husband and wife. Remember, we are to become "one flesh" (Genesis 2:24). These secular ideas are contrary to the perfect design for marriage, in which a wife's role *is* dependent on the husband's. However, as with all other aspects of God's perfect will for us, we fall short. When we find ourselves in an enmeshed relationship that is functioning outside of God's plan, we are living in sin. What is this specific sin and how do we overcome it?

While the abuser's primary outward sin is violence and abusiveness, his inward sin is anger and pride. For the abused, the primary sin is idolatry, and the outward manifestation is her worship of her abusive husband and being unequally yoked. Whether we are in an abusive relationship or a healthy relationship, any form of idolatry is sinful and damaging to ourselves and our partners. Secular counseling theories would tell us that when one remains in an abusive relationship, codependency is a likely factor in the victim's decision. However, in the abusive relationship in which the victim is a Christian, the "codependency" is manifested either through the misuse of Scripture (which has been addressed and will continue to be addressed in the next chapter), and/or through the sin of idolatry. How do we recognize spousal idolatry?

Jesus said, as recorded in Matthew 10:25, "If the head of the house has been called Beelzebub, how much more the members of his household!" Beelzebub is another name for Satan. We know from previous Bible study and discussion that the "head of the house" in God's perfect design is man. From this we gather that the man leads the family. However, as in the above Scripture, sometimes he leads his family to death.* However, the family does not have to follow. Indeed, spiritually, it is impossible for them to follow and still be within God's will, unless they believe living in sin is God's will. When a husband is not fulfilling his godly leadership role, his wife is torn between following him and following God. Although slightly out of context, 1 Corinthians 10:21 can apply here. It says:

---

*The application of this Scripture here is admittedly out of context. However, it is my contention that the spiritual principle implied by Jesus is the same whether in its original context or a context of family abuse.

You cannot drink the cup of the Lord and the cup of demons too; you cannot have a part of both the Lord's table and the table of demons.

Likewise, Jesus says in another passage that "he who is not with me is against me" (Matthew 12:30). In Christian homes where domestic violence is occurring, a definite spiritual division develops. To the family who is experiencing this, it is evident that the house is divided. However, for the outsider, the spiritual division may not be apparent. Perhaps the biggest mistake a pastor or other church member makes when counseling a couple with issues of abuse in the marriage is to assume that the abused and abuser are spiritually on equal footing. This is especially true if the abuser presents for counseling during the "honeymoon" phase of the cycle. He may seem genuinely repentant, and the depth of the sin may appear less severe than it actually is. Perhaps it is so subtle that it does not seem like sin at all. Maybe you are wondering if you are living with an abusive spouse.

Remember we discussed the reasons why Christian women stay in abusive relationships. One of those reasons was that we should not judge one another. The discussion centered on the biblical point that judgment can be construed as discernment. That is why God told us that "the spiritual man makes judgments about all things, but he himself is not subject to any man's judgment" (1 Corinthians 2:15). How do we make judgments, and, more specifically, how does someone who suspects abuse in a relationship make a judgment? Our carnal nature would tell us to look first at what the person says about who he is. However, we must be very careful. Perhaps the abuser claims his faith. That is not enough to ensure safety in the relationship. Titus 1:16 tells about deceivers, "they claim to know God but by their actions they deny him." We should examine the outward actions of a person to determine their faith, but, this type of evidence is valid only if a discrepancy occurs between stated and actual behavior. An abusive spouse can often appear very loving toward the abused spouse. In these instances discernment requires a greater test of evidence. Jesus gives the following warning in Matthew 7:15-16:

Watch out for false prophets. They come to you in sheep's clothing, but inwardly they are ferocious wolves. By their fruit you will recognize them.

Outside appearances can be very deceptive. One of Satan's strategies is to look like a sheep so he can sneak in with the sheep unnoticed, but his real intention is to harm them. The *only* way to know if someone is a sheep or a wolf is to look for the fruit in his or her life. The fruit of the Spirit is listed in Galatians 5:22-23:

But the fruit of the Spirit is love, joy, peace, patience, kindness, goodness, faithfulness, gentleness and self-control.

We must discern the evidence of these virtues in people's lives, including our own. All of these may not be evident at one time. Even if lacking, we would not necessarily conclude that the Spirit is missing. However, if several fruits are absent, or one "branch" in particular bears bad fruit, we should proceed with caution. The book of 1 John provides further "testing ground" for discerning spirits. Just by reviewing the list of fruits, without even knowing the particulars of a situation, we may see implications of an abusive spouse. The big red flag would probably be in the area of self-control, but it may be in all of the areas listed, as they are interrelated. It is difficult to continue to be abusive and have evidence of the Spirit in your life, just as it is difficult to remain in an abusive relationship without falling into the sin of idolatry.

Now that we know the specific sin often committed by an abused spouse is idolatry, we need to understand this sin as it relates to God's word. Luke 4:8 tells us to "Worship the Lord your God and serve Him only" (see also Deuteronomy 6:13 and 10:20). What exactly does it mean to worship? 1 Corinthians 7:23 states,

You were bought at a price; do not become slaves of men.

Paul's focus in chapter seven seems to be marriage, and even though he appears to diverge to a discussion on slavery, he remains within a context of marriage throughout the chapter. The original

Greek word for slave, or *doulos,* in the above Scripture, is defined as "one who gives himself up to another's will" and "devoted to another to the disregard of one's own interests." Both of these expounded interpretations apply directly to the sin of idolatry within the abusive marriage, and both of these definitions allude to a degree of worship. The abused spouse quite often remains in the relationship because of her sense of devotion, even when she knows her devotion may be fatal.

Another aspect of worship can be understood by Jesus' statement: "Anyone who loves his father or mother more than me is not worthy of me" (Matthew 10:37). This same Scripture can also apply to the husband-wife relationship. The Lord is not saying that a husband and wife should not love each other. Rather, an abused wife may love her husband to such a degree and manner that it is more than she loves even the Lord. This is the core of her idolatry. She loves her husband with the fervor and addiction that she should reserve for the Lord. Deuteronomy 6:5 gives us what Jesus called the "greatest commandment" (Matthew 22:37): "Love the Lord your God with *all* your heart and with all your soul and with all your strength." Notice the strong qualifiers here: with *all* your heart, soul, and strength. We are to love the Lord like that. He does not say to love our husbands, our wives, or even our children like that. He tells us that He is the only one who deserves our fervent love. Remember, He is the one who gave us that love to begin with. It is a sacred love.

Jesus said, as recorded in Matthew 7:6, "Do not give dogs what is sacred; do not throw your pearls to pigs. If you do they may trample them under their feet, and then turn and tear you to pieces." This requires a degree of discernment. We may find biblical assistance in our discernment when we look at 1 Corinthians 13: 4-8, which gives us a deeper definition of the kind of love we are to have for one another. However, this same portion of biblical text also serves as a "measuring stick" for the kind of love our spouses demonstrate toward us. "Love is not easily angered, it keeps no record of wrongs." The love of an abusive spouse is irreconcilable with the love God describes in this passage. God's plan for marriage is clearly not established in the abusive marriage. The abused wife is perverting the 1 Corinthians definition of love toward her husband in that she is forsaking God in the process.

Some may argue that God is glorified through such an example of love. However, Scripture also tells us that we are the temple of God (Acts 17:24, 1 Corinthians 3:16, 1 Corinthians 6:19, 2 Corinthians 6:16). Allowing God's temple to be beaten is an act of desecration. In this same way, when we love someone else the way God asks us to exclusively love Him, we not only become a slave to the person we think we are loving, we are also committing the sin of idolatry.

Now that we understand the abused spouse's accountability in terms of the sin of idolatry, what are the next steps in the relationship? As with any sin, repentance is required for one to be released from the bondage of the sin. The abused wife must refocus herself onto the Lord. Once she has regained her strength in the Lord enough to entrust her life to Him, she must attempt to reconcile the relationship. The only way reconciliation can occur is if the abusive spouse also takes accountability for the sin. Several Scriptures give us a model for dealing with others' sins (Matthew 18:15-17, Ephesians 5:11, Titus 3:9). The abused spouse must begin talking about the abuse if she has not already. Domestic violence is a shameful secret that many women hide. Darkness must give way to the light. She may seek counsel from the pastor or other church members. If that is the case, the counselor needs to consult with elders in the church to form a group of at least two who will confront the abusive spouse, if that spouse claims his faith and/or membership in the church. This may lead to greater danger for the abused spouse, so extreme caution should be taken. If she suffers severe physical abuse, confrontation may lead to retaliation. A psychological perspective gives a couple of reasons for this, but the spiritual perspective is that the battle line has now been drawn and the war has been waged.

Chapter 17

The Believer and Divorce

Now that we have a better understanding of the accountability that each partner in an abusive relationship shares for the abuse, we must discuss what happens when the abusive partner fails to accept accountability, and the unity of the relationship becomes spiritually severed. If the abusive partner accepts accountability, then the relationship can begin to heal and the husband and wife may have the chance to reconcile. Often, when the abused woman accepts accountability and adopts a leadership position within the family unit, the abuse worsens. This is because one of the abuser's primary motives is control. When the abused partner begins to take control in the relationship, the spiritual battle between the two of them will intensify. The abused spouse may be hurt and confused about what steps to take next. Perhaps she has prayed endlessly, fasted, anointed her surroundings with oil, sought counseling, been baptized, has deidolized her husband, and studied God's word. She has faithfully pursued all of these spiritual activities, and the abuse worsens.

Immediately getting away from the abuser is the first, and most critical, step. It may also be the hardest one. However the abused spouse chooses to leave is based on circumstance, timing, and God's protection. Most states have some sort of protection order, which legally keeps the abuser away from his victim. This avenue has many advantages. First, it allows legal protection from further harm to the abused spouse and/or the children. Second, it allows the marital relationship to remain legally intact. A protection order is not final, nor is it even recognized unless the filing spouse chooses to use it. In other words, she must not only obtain the order, but also call the police to implement it. Although a restraining order prohibits either spouse from having any contact, most spouses attempt communication of some sort, so reconciliation can still occur if both partners are willing. Third, it provides both spouses a safe cooling off period. Both spouses can more effectively concentrate on God, and allow Him to work in their lives because the spiritual friction is diminished. In less lethal relationships, a protection order does allow the police to make an arrest if the abuser attempts to contact, harass, or further abuse the people protected by the order. This may send a strong and effective message to some abusers that the abused spouse is finally holding them accountable for their abusiveness. The protection order, or even a mutual agreement to separate, may be the ideal way to address violence within a relationship and begin the process of healing. The disadvantage of the protection order is that the order itself is merely a piece of paper, and will not provide any guarantee of physical protection. A protection order will not stop a bullet. Experience shows that most women separate from their abusive spouses on the average of three times before they finally choose to completely sever the relationship. As was the case of Alicia, some women must flee and completely sever the relationship in order to stay alive. For other women, legal issues must be addressed in a court of family law, and the protection order is not sufficient for settling or protecting the legal interests of the abused spouse. For many women, a protection order is simply not enough to cause the abuser to repent.

What options does a woman have when she has done everything legally, physically, emotionally, and even spiritually possible to stop the abuse in her life, but it continues? One option, which is often unthinkable within the church, is divorce. The purpose here is not to advocate that abused spouses divorce their abusers. The purpose is to study the entirety of God's own words on the matter, to offer a scriptural basis to those who believe God has called them out of their abusive marriages, and to challenge those who consider divorce always to be against God's will. The place to start a discussion on God's specific will is to define God's general will.

Some theologians have defined two distinct types of God's will. The first is the sovereign will of God. It is God's ultimate will. It is the highest standard. It is characterized by the perfection to which God calls us. This is also the part of God's will we often fail to live up to. An example of this sovereign will of God is found in the first section of this book, where God's design for marriage is mapped out. God's example given to us through the account of pre-sin Adam and Eve is His sovereign will for our marriages. This type of God's will may also be characterized as the general will of God. It is the will of God that remains the same across the board, for all people.

The second will of God is His permissive will. This form of God's will is specific. That is, it is tailor-made for our individual lives. The permissive will of God allows sin in our lives. It gives "permission" for sin to be in our lives because it is always based on God's glory. In other words, even if it is not God's perfect will, God allows it because it will ultimately bring glory to Him. Our sin is not acceptable simply because it is included as part of God's purpose for our life. Wrong is never made right in the permissive will of God. However, in the permissive will of God, "wrong" is not only allowed, it is used for God's ultimate purpose. The distinction is the difference between acceptance and allowance. We are still held accountable for the sin, but God allows the sin to happen and even to continue so that it may eventually bring glory to Him. This logical theology reconciles God's stated will with the reality of our sinfulness, while still maintaining the sovereignty of God. However, another idea presented by theologians is that God maintains complete sovereignty over all things. In other words, we have free will only within the circumstances God ordains, and His foreknowledge facilitates the circumstances. In relation to divorce in the Christian marriage, there are Scriptures that support both views.

The entire book of Deuteronomy outlines God's laws, rules, and commands concerning the Israelites. This portion of Scripture is called the Mosaic Law (the Law of Moses). Chapters 21 through 23 address the laws concerning marriage and family life. Divorce is mentioned in Deuteronomy 22:19 and 29. It is mentioned in a context that indicates it is forbidden. However, when we read the entirety of the passage, we clearly see that the prohibition for the man to divorce the woman is a part of his punishment for either giving the woman a bad name, or for violating her. The punishment for his sins is that he must marry her and may never divorce her. Is not marriage supposed to be a blessing ordained by God? Why is the marriage, and the law against ending it, a punishment in this case? In Old Testament times wives were often recognized as a commodity, but also as a burden. The decision to marry was not always based on love. It was frequently based on social standards and customs. The number of wives, concubines, and maidservants a man had were signs of his wealth. That was not necessarily the social milieu of the Israelites, but of other cultures. However, for the Israelites, to be married for any reason other than love was a burden because custom dictated, much as it does today, that the man was responsible to care financially for his wife. For the Israelites, it was a great burden to have a wife who was not loved. The punishment for specific sins committed toward a woman was marriage with no allowance for divorce.

Divorce is also mentioned in Deuteronomy 24:1-4. Here, the Mosaic Law not only allowed for divorce, it specified that a certificate was to be issued in the event of a divorce, and if the divorced woman remarries, she cannot return to marry the first husband. The grounds for divorce are based on the man's displeasure when he finds something indecent about his wife. Why would God allow for divorce in Old Testament times? Jesus Himself tells us, as recorded in Matthew 19:8:

> Moses permitted you to divorce your wives because your hearts were hard. But it was not this way from the beginning.

Divorce was allowed in Old Testament times because the Israelites had hardened hearts toward their spouses. This could be interpreted as the permissive will of God, because Malachi 2:16 tells us God's feelings about divorce:

> "I hate divorce," says the Lord God of Israel.

Either God is contradicting Himself, or we need to gain further understanding. We discussed the Malachi verse previously in the context of the historical and biblical record of abuse within marriage. Divorce was allowed because of hard-heartedness and abuse. God Himself issued a certificate of divorce to His faithless wife, Israel, because of her spiritual adultery or idolatry (Jeremiah 3:8). Although Israel was later reconciled to God, it seems that divorce was a God-ordained response to sin, and facilitated repentance and reconciliation (Jeremiah 3: 12-25).

The first New Testament Scripture concerning divorce is recorded in Matthew 5:31-32:

> It has been said, "Anyone who divorces his wife must give her a certificate of divorce." But I tell you that anyone who divorces his wife, except for marital unfaithfulness, causes her to become an adulteress, and anyone who marries the divorced woman commits adultery.

A slightly different version of this teaching is recorded in Mark 10:1-12:

> Anyone who divorces his wife and marries another woman commits adultery against her. And if she divorces her husband and marries another man, she commits adultery.

God is so awesome throughout His word! Two of Jesus' disciples recorded the exact same sermon and each had a different perspective on what was taught. In the first verse the sin is attributed to the woman and her potential new husband. What happened to the accountability of the first husband who divorces his wife? Does he not sin if he divorces his wife? Upon closer examination, Jesus implies that the actual sin of divorce, as recorded through this verse, originates with the husband who divorces his wife. This is because he "causes her" to sin. God is attributing the cause of the wife's sin to the husband. Remember the husband's duty toward his wife is to "make her holy, cleansing her by the washing with water through the word, and to present her to himself as a radiant church, without stain or wrinkle or any other blemish, but holy and blameless" (Ephesians 5:26-27). Divorcing her would be causing her to sin, and thus he himself is sinning by not fulfilling his godly duty in the marriage.

Mark's verse provides a mutual accountability and sharing of the burden of sin in the event of a divorce. Another distinction between Matthew's and Mark's versions of Jesus' sermon at Perea is that in the first verse Jesus gives an "exception clause" that is absent in the second verse. This exception clause is often interpreted and applied by Christians in a legalistic and inappropriate manner. It is often taken literally to mean that divorce is not allowed unless one spouse has committed adultery, but the verse does not actually say that. It says "marital unfaithfulness." The King James Version of the same verse translates the term as "fornication." The actual Greek word is *porneia,* from which we get our word "pornography." Sexual sin is the most common biblical translation of the word *porneia.* It is usually translated as a specific sexual sin, such as homosexuality or adultery. In the Matthew verse it is not translated literally as adultery, but as marital unfaithfulness. Interestingly, *porneia* has also been used as a metaphor for the worship of idols in other Scriptures (particularly in Revelation). This could apply in a loose interpretation. If applied to this teaching, then marital unfaithfulness could include all things related to idol worship. As discussed in the last chapter, domestic violence falls within this category.

Some conservative teachers might argue that Jesus' original intention was to make a divorce exception only when actual adultery occurred. A counterargument could question a legalistic interpretation by using Jesus' teaching on adultery. In Matthew 5:28 Jesus says, "But I tell you that anyone who looks at a woman lustfully has already committed adultery with her in his heart." The Lord looks at our hearts when He makes a judgment. Therefore, some believe that this "exception" in Matthew's record is not really an exception for divorce. Matthew's gospel is primarily written for the Jews, which may explain why the "exception clause" is not found in any of the other gospels. The Jewish custom dictated a betrothal period, which was similar to the modern Western engagement. One major difference between engagement and betrothal is that betrothal was seen as legally binding. It was mandatory for the

Jewish people to marry a virgin (Leviticus 21:14). Therefore, if a man or woman had sexual relations with someone other than their betrothed during the betrothal period, this caused a dilemma. Matthew's record may alleviate this dilemma by allowing the slighted Jewish man or woman to "divorce" the betrothed without committing a sin. Once married there was no exception for divorce.

The "certificate of divorce" that Moses spoke of, and which is still a factor of our legal and recordkeeping system, is an allowance by God. It has never been God's expressed will for a man and woman to divorce. From God's point of view, a man and woman can be divorced in their hearts long before they actually divorce, because God does not consider the piece of paper; He cares about our hearts. In fact, Jesus said God allowed divorce to occur in the first place because "your hearts were hard." Even so, for those who feel more comfortable with a common interpretation of the Matthew and Mark verses on divorce, in both verses Jesus implies that the actual sin of divorce is not committed until the spouses remarry, and then it is a sin of adultery. There is no indication that divorce itself is a sin. The sin comes from the second marriage or, rather, from the sexual encounters that would occur in a second marriage.

An even more conservatively interpreted teaching on divorce was given by Paul in 1 Corinthians 7:10-17. The entire chapter deals with marriage and divorce, but verses 10-17 particularly relate to our study because it is the only teaching in the Bible on spiritually mixed marriages. First, Paul writes in verses 10 and 11: "A wife must not separate from her husband. *But if she does,* she must remain unmarried or else be reconciled to her husband" (italics added). Paul more directly states Jesus' own implication from the previous verses. In other words, it is best not to divorce, but if divorce occurs, remarriage is forbidden. Paul continues in verses 12 through 17 to write about the spiritually mixed marriage. Notice that he is careful to point out in verse 12 that this teaching is his, and not necessarily the Lord's: "To the rest I say this (I, not the Lord)." This is contrary to verse 10 in which Paul qualifies the teaching on divorce as being a command from the Lord.

To summarize Paul's teaching on spiritually mixed marriages, he writes that a Christian must remain married to his or her unbelieving spouse. In verse 15 he also writes that if the unbelieving spouse wants to leave, "let him do so." Therefore, the believing spouse is no longer "bound" in such a circumstance. He further writes, "God has called us to live in peace." Paul recognizes that a spiritual battle is inevitable when a believer and unbeliever live under the same roof. Paul's teaching on spiritually mixed marriages assumes that the believing spouse was saved after the marriage took place. God is against spiritually mixed relationships (Deuteronomy 22:10, 1 Corinthians 5:9-10, 1 Corinthians 7:39, 2 Corinthians 6:14-16, Ephesians 5:6-7). It is contrary to Scripture for a believer to marry an unbeliever, so Paul addresses what a believer is to do if saved after the marriage has occurred. Even so, Paul specifically stated that this teaching was from him, and not from the Lord. Jesus himself taught against legalism. God is most concerned with our hearts. What does a husband or wife do when one or both of their hearts are hard toward each other?

We know that God can and does miraculously change people. There is no question of faith here. However, sometimes God chooses not to miraculously change people, at least not in the way we hope that He will. We see from the example in Exodus 7:3 that God hardened Pharaoh's heart for the purpose of bringing His people out of Egypt. Why God did not accomplish this by softening Pharaoh's heart, and having Pharaoh just let them go peacefully, we do not know for certain ("Therefore God has mercy on whom he wants to have mercy, and he hardens whom he wants to harden," Romans 9:18). We do know that the hardness of Pharaoh's heart caused many events that had spiritual significance. These events would not have occurred if Pharaoh's heart was not hard. Through this example we see that "in all things God works for the good of those who love Him" (Romans 8:28).

This story alludes to the concepts of the sovereign and permissive wills of God. The hardening of Pharaoh's heart may not have been the sovereign will of God, but it certainly was the permissive will of God. Whether it be the abused spouse, the abusive spouse, or both spouses whose hearts are hard within the marital relationship, God can soften or harden them according to His ultimate purpose. In other words, while we know that God's sovereign will is for Christians never to divorce, we also know that God's permissive will may sometimes allow for divorce in Christian marriages. Why would God allow divorce?

We do not always know what God's purpose may be. In fact, most times we will not know beforehand what God's purpose is. A fitting example of this is found in the story of Abraham and Isaac, as recorded in Genesis 21. Abraham had prayed for a son for decades. God finally blessed him with Isaac when Abraham was 100 years old. We also know from chapter 22, verse 1 that God tested Abraham. Abraham had prayed for a son for so long that when Isaac finally came, Abraham began to worship Isaac within his heart, and had forgotten to worship the God who had faithfully kept His promise. So, God spoke to Abraham, telling him to sacrifice his only son Isaac as a burnt offering. Abraham faithfully obeyed and made the three-day journey to the top of the mountain, where God told him to sacrifice Isaac. This may seem strange. Keep in mind that in Old Testament times people made sacrificial offerings to the Lord for their sins. This story also serves as a prophetic example of the love of our Father and the sacrifice of His only Son for us. God, knowing that Abraham began to worship Isaac, asked Abraham to sacrifice his son in order that He may test him. Abraham set out to obey God's command, unsure of the real purpose. In that long and painful three-day journey, Abraham had to have his heart cleansed of Isaac. By the time Abraham reached the top of that mountain with Isaac, he had dethroned his son and returned God to the rightful place in his heart. Abraham passed the test and God spared Isaac.

This story is not only an awesome historical account of the father of Israel, it is also a God-inspired metaphor for His purpose in our own lives. Sometimes we, like Abraham, become so in love with people that we begin to worship them. Sometimes God asks us to sacrifice those relationships. When we look at Abraham and Isaac's story from this perspective, it would be preposterous to imagine Abraham refusing to obey God's command. For in doing so, even though Abraham may not have clearly understood at the time, he would have been harming himself. God's will, whether permissive or sovereign, is always working for our best interest.

Many pastors, church leaders, and counselors believe that divorce is never God's will. These same people would not consider the account of Abraham and Isaac an example of the calling God may have on our own marriages, but that calling is possible, if not literally, perhaps spiritually. If God asked Abraham to sacrifice his own son, an eagerly awaited promise, it is possible that He would ask an abused wife to sacrifice her marital relationship (whether literally or in spirit) in order that He may retain the rightful place of worship in her heart. If, and that is a cautious "if," she receives that calling from God and ignores it, she is living in sin. I say "if" cautiously because I recognize that some would find this teaching to be inaccurate and out of context. However, our personal relationship with God is just that; it is so personal that it is inviolable to anyone else. If an abused spouse feels God has called her out of her marriage then no one has the right to make judgment or look down on her, nor does she have to live in condemnation for obeying such a calling.

Unfortunately, a literal application of Scripture may lead to a denunciation of the permissive will of God in some cases. In the abusive Christian marriage, a few Scriptures speak God's permissive will to the abused spouse. One such Scripture is found in 2 Corinthians 6:14-16:

> Do not be yoked together with unbelievers. For what do righteousness and wickedness have in common? Or what fellowship can light have with darkness? What harmony is there between Christ and Belial? What does a believer have in common with an unbeliever? What agreement is there between the temple of God and idols? For *we are the temple of the living God* (italics added).

This Scripture is important in reference to the abusive marriage. The first reason is obvious. We are not to be unequally yoked. Although Paul taught on unequally yoked marriages (1 Corinthians 7:10-17), as we previously discussed, he sets apart his own instructions from the Lord's in this passage. The second part of this verse, which is crucial to the context of family violence, is that we are the temple of God. The Holy Spirit resides in us. As such, to allow ourselves to willingly and knowingly be abused is the same as if we allowed someone to desecrate God's temple building structure. It is a sin of blasphemy. Furthermore, Jesus tells us in Matthew 18:8,

> If your hand or your foot causes you to sin, cut it off and throw it away. It is better for you to enter life maimed or crippled than to have two hands or two feet and be thrown into the eternal fire.

One cannot continue abusive behaviors and continue to serve God. As long as the abuser serves pride and anger, there is spiritual division in the home. When one spouse goes astray, the other is forced to make a choice of whom to serve, and when the straying spouse is the spiritual leader, the following spouse is probably living in sin. Often the church, whether literally or through implication, brings condemnation onto the abused spouse because he or she has made a decision to leave the marriage. A recent trend in some churches is toward compassionate counsel of abused women, but the church is still a long way from acknowledging the plight of the abused husband. Indeed, the spiritual dynamics and counsel are very different for the abused husband.

We have examined what the Bible says specifically about divorce, and we have a better understanding of Scriptures that could be applied and used to substantiate God's permissive will for an abused spouse to divorce the abuser. The rest is up to God. If you are in or have been in an abusive relationship, then be confident that whatever conviction God gives to you is His specific will for your life. No one can stand between you and God on that. If you are unsure about what to do, seek, study, and pray. God will speak to you. You are to "obey God rather than men" (Acts 5:29).

If you counsel or know someone who is in an abusive marriage, then you hopefully have a better understanding of how to use Scripture to support and encourage the battered spouse, and are prevented from condemning the abused spouse further. Divorce, whether in the heart, on paper, or both, is a severing of the unity of the marital relationship. It is extremely painful, and is most certainly not an easy decision.

Teachers in the church will often quote a 1999 study by the Barna Research Group, which showed that 24 percent of non-Christians, and 27 percent of Christians report having been divorced—a statistically significant difference.* A misperception in church leadership is that divorce, because it is common, is an easy solution too readily applied to minor problems within a marriage. That could not be further from the truth.

One study showed that 19 percent of divorced women reported they divorced their husbands because of violence (Kurz,1996). How many of those who cited violence as a reason for divorce were Christians? Furthermore, a 1986 study of batterers in treatment showed that more than 44.6 percent claimed to be Protestant, and 33.7 percent claimed to be Catholic (Hamberger and Hastings, 1986). Collectively, that is more than 75 percent of batterers who claim to have a religious affiliation! It would be interesting to know the real reasons why the divorce rate is higher in the Christian community.

> And everyone who has left houses or brothers or sisters or father or mother or children or fields for my sake will receive a hundred times as much and will inherit eternal life (Matthew 19:29).

---

*The Barna study made several errors in research methodology and grossly failed to share confounding variables to the data. For example, the study did not clarify if those Christians who reported having been divorced were divorced prior to or after a religious conversion. They also broadly defined "born-again Christians" to include groups who have vague and even unbiblical beliefs. Furthermore, they failed to research the reasons why divorce occurs. That is relevant and important information for an audience that is trying to solve the divorce problem, and it quite possibly would reveal different reasons for the Christian and non-Christian.

Chapter 18

Rewards of Faithfulness: The Redemption of Ruth

The book of Ruth, a mere four chapters, is not only a historical account of a woman named Ruth and her faithfulness to God, but also a profound lesson of hope for all believers. Most Bible scholars, theologians, and pastors see the book as a prophetic glimpse of our salvation through Jesus Christ. To the abused spouse, Ruth offers more than just salvation. Her story offers redemption, restoration, and hope for a "right" marital relationship.

Ruth's story begins with a Hebrew family who fled from Bethlehem-Judah to a foreign land because of a famine in their own land. The family, steeped in the faith of its forefathers, leaves the land of blessing to go to a land less favored by God. This family, Elimelech, his wife Naomi, and his two sons Mahlon and Kilion, make their journey to the land of Moab, where Elimelech subsequently dies. This foreign land, Moab, is referred to in Psalm 108:9 as God's "washpot." About ten years later, both Mahlon and Kilion marry Moabite wives. Ruth, a Moabitess, is taken in marriage by Elimelech's son Mahlon. While still in the land of Moab, both of Naomi's sons die, leaving their wives widows. Naomi is now widowed in a foreign land without her sons, and she finds herself alone. Naomi then seems to understand that following her husband out of Bethlehem-Judah was an act of faithlessness toward God, and she makes a decision to return to her homeland, which she heard had recovered from the famine. She urges her young daughters-in-law to remain in Moab to remarry men of their own nationality. Orpah decides she is going to stay in Moab, as Naomi suggested, but Ruth struggles with the prospect of losing her mother-in-law. Orpah's decision was to turn away from the laws, traditions, and faith of Naomi and her people—to turn back to the ways of her idolatrous country. Ruth, however, makes a pledge to Naomi when she says, "Don't urge me to leave you or to turn back from you. Where you go I will go, and where you stay I will stay. Your people will be my people and your God my God. Where you die I will die, and there I will be buried. May the Lord deal with me, be it ever so severely, if anything but death separates you and me" (Ruth 1:16-17). Ruth was very committed to her mother-in-law, and also toward her God. That meant possible discrimination and social segregation for Ruth, as she would be a foreigner, a pagan, in the land of Naomi's heritage. Not only was Ruth an outsider, she was a widow, which made remarriage highly unlikely as the faithful Hebrew people did not marry foreign women. Ruth, fully prepared to remain without a husband the rest of her life, vows to remain faithful to her mother-in-law.

Naomi and Ruth make the 120-mile journey from Moab to Bethlehem-Judah. This is a prodigal journey for Naomi, who admitted that the Lord had afflicted her during her years in Moab (Ruth 1:20-21). Naomi and Ruth arrive in Bethlehem-Judah during the barley harvest, both destitute and empty-handed. Ruth then makes the acquaintance of Boaz, a wealthy landowner in the region. A Levitical custom was for landowners to leave the corners of their land unharvested, so the poor and foreign could glean after the landowner and his harvesters had (Leviticus 19:9-10). Naomi and Ruth being poor, Ruth asks Naomi if she may go and glean corn for the two of them. Naomi grants Ruth permission, and Ruth happens onto some land owned by Boaz. Boaz visits his reapers and takes notice of Ruth gleaning in his field. He asks about her, and then Boaz not only invites Ruth to stay in his field, he asks the men in the field not to touch her (Ruth 2:9). Ruth falls to her feet in humility for the kindness that Boaz has shown her, and he in turn treats her as his own. Upon returning to Naomi after the day's gathering, Ruth discovers the true identity of Boaz.

A Levitical custom, later to be incorporated into the Law of Moses, was for the brother, or nearest kin of the deceased man, to marry his widow (Genesis 38:8, Deuteronomy 25:5-10). This was seen as a necessary act of redemption for the deceased man and his lineage. Boaz was a kin of Elimelech (Ruth 2:1), which is why Naomi called Boaz "one of our kinsman-redeemers" (Ruth 2:20). Under the Mosaic Law, Boaz was not only free, but obligated to marry Ruth. There was, however, a kin closer in relation than Boaz. Boaz, being the fair man that he was, gave this other kin an opportunity to redeem Elimelech's property and family. This man wanted no part of the redemption, as it meant acquiring the responsibility for the women. Boaz, who was very much in love with Ruth, married her and they conceived a son (Ruth 4:13). The son of Ruth and Boaz was Obed, the father of Jesse, the father of David. We also know that through the lineage of Boaz and Ruth, Jesus Christ was born (Matthew 1:1-16).

What a wonderful story of love and redemption! Many scholars believe that Boaz is a foreshadowing of Jesus Christ, our own kinsman-redeemer or *goel*. However, had it not been Ruth's faithfulness and trust in her mother-in-law, she never would have made acquaintance with Boaz. Ruth's relationship with Naomi is very much like our relationship with Jesus Christ. When we follow Him out of a known land, and in humility accept whatever consequences ensue, we are ultimately blessed! Likewise, Naomi had traveled to a foreign land, a land of pagans and idolaters, with her husband and sons. She was widowed and abandoned in that land, and like the prodigal son, returned home to her own people. Had it not been for her prodigal journey, as well as the loss of her family, she may not have shared in the blessing of redemption nor been a part of the lineage that bore the King of Israel and, later, the Son of God. Ruth herself was blessed, because God replaced her first husband, Mahlon (literally meaning "sick"), with a man who was more than just a husband, but a redeemer who deeply loved and protected her.

Sometimes, in the midst of trials and human suffering, it is difficult for us to see the bigger picture. God's ways are mysterious to us at times (Job 36:26), and His ways are always higher than our own (Isaiah 55:9). God's word gives many examples of people who suffered, some seeming unjust, because God had a plan of redemption. He tears down, but also builds up; He injures, but also heals (Job 5:18). "And we know that in all things God works for the good of those who love Him, who have been called according to His purpose" (Romans 8:28). Another beautiful Scripture that we can meditate on while in the midst of trials and warfare is Jeremiah 29:11:

> "For I know the plans I have for you," declares the Lord, "plans to prosper you and not to harm you, plans to give you hope and a future. Then you will call upon me and come and pray to me, and I will listen to you. You will seek me and find me when you seek me with all your heart."

Another example is found in the story of Joseph (Genesis chapters 37-50). After many trials and losses, Joseph, a foreigner in the land of Egypt, and a former slave, is raised up to be the head over all of Egypt. He then surmises that the past years of his life were all for God's bigger plan, which was to save his family from the famine of their own land (Genesis 45:7-8).

We also read in the account of Job that while Job was severely afflicted, God blessed him with twice as much of everything He had allowed Satan to take (Job 42:10). Job's example is an important one in understanding Satan's working in our own lives, because even though Job's losses were at the hand of Satan, Satan could do nothing without God's permission first. In fact, God suggested Job to Satan (Job 1:8).

We see a similar confession by the apostle Paul, when he tells us that in order to keep him "from becoming conceited," Satan gave him a "thorn in his flesh" (2 Corinthians 12:7).

We can rest assured as Christians that our suffering is never in vain. James writes,

> Blessed is the man who perseveres under trial, because when he has stood the test, he will receive the crown of life that God has promised to those who love Him (James 1:12).

Perhaps you are reading this and do not feel blessed. Perhaps you are counseling someone who is experiencing spousal abuse, and he or she does not feel blessed. Remember that our faith transcends our feelings. Whether a decision is made to remain in the abusive relationship, or to leave the relationship, even if temporarily, there are bound to be periods of difficulty and discomfort. Even still, we can fix our eyes on Jesus! As the apostle Paul so eloquently wrote in 2 Corinthians 4:7-18:

> But we have this treasure in jars of clay to show that this all-surpassing power is from God and not from us. We are hard pressed on every side, but not crushed; perplexed, but not in despair; persecuted, but not abandoned; struck down, but not destroyed. We always carry around in our body the death of Jesus, so that the life of Jesus may also be revealed in our body. For we who are alive are always being given over to death for Jesus' sake, so that his life may be revealed in our mortal body. So then, death is at work in us, but life is at work in you. It is written: "I believed; therefore, I have spoken." With that same spirit of faith we also believe and therefore speak, because we know that the one who raised the Lord Jesus from the dead will also raise us with Jesus and present us with you in his presence. All this is for your benefit, so that the grace that is reaching more and more people may cause thanksgiving to overflow to the glory of God. Therefore we do not lose heart. Though outwardly we are wasting away, yet inwardly we are being renewed day by day. For our light and momentary troubles are achieving for us an eternal glory that far outweighs them all. So we fix our eyes not on what is seen, but on what is unseen. For what is seen is temporary, but what is unseen is eternal.

> Still another said, "I will follow you, Lord; but first let me go back and say good-by to my family." Jesus replied, "No one who puts his hand to the plow and looks back is fit for service in the kingdom of God" (Luke 9:61-62).

References

Bachman, Ronet and Saltzman, Linda (1995). "Violence Against Women: Estimates from the Redesigned Survey." *Bureau of Justice Statistics: Special Report* (August).

Barna, George (1999). "Christians Are More Likely to Experience Divorce Than Are Non-Christians." Barna Research Online (December 21). <http://www.barna.org/cgibin/PagePressRelease.asp?PressReleaseID=39&Reference=C>.

Barnett, O.W., Keyson, M., and Thelen, R.E. (1992). "Women's Violence As a Response to Male Abuse." Paper presented at the 100th Annual Convention of the American Psychological Association, Washington, DC, August.

Brookoff, Daniel (1997). "Drugs, Alcohol, and Domestic Violence in Memphis." *National Institute of Justice: Research Preview* (October).

Federal Bureau of Investigation. *Uniform Crime Reports* (1992). Washington, DC.

Grady, J. Lee (2001). "Control Freaks and the Women Who Love Them." *New Man* (January/February), pp. 40-44.

Hamberger, Kevin and Hastings, James (1986). "Characteristics of Spouse Abusers: Predictors of Treatment Acceptance." *Journal of Interpersonal Violence* 1(3): 363-373.

Henry, Matthew (2000). *Matthew Henry's Complete Commentary on the Whole Bible: Complete and Unabridged.* Eleventh Printing. Peabody, MA: Hendrickson Publishers.

Kurz, D. (1996). "Separation, Divorce, and Woman Abuse." *Violence Against Women* 2(1): 63-81.

Random House Dictionary of the English Language, Second Edition, Unabridged. (1987). New York: Random House.

Strong's Concordance with Hebrew and Greek Lexicon (Online). <http://www.eliyah.com/lexicon.html>.

Tjaden, Patricia (1997). "The Crime of Stalking: How Big is the Problem?" *National Institute of Justice: Research Preview* (November).

Today's Parallel Bible: NIV, NAS, KJV, NLT (2000). Grand Rapids. MI: Zondervan.

Additional Resources

Please note that inclusion of the following resources does not constitute endorsement of any beliefs or ideas expressed by the individual organizations represented here. These are general resources available for further information and/or help.

Alcoholics for Christ
1216 N. Campbell Rd.
Royal Oak, MI 48067
800-441-7877
http://www.alcoholicsforchrist.com

Center for the Prevention of Sexual and Domestic Violence
2400 North 45th St. #10
Seattle, WA 98103
206-634-1903
http://www.cpsdv.org

Christians for Biblical Equality
122 West Franklin Ave. Suite 218
Minneapolis, MN 55404-2451
612-872-6898
http://www.cbeinternational.org

Council on Biblical Manhood and Womanhood
2825 Lexington Road, Box 926
Louisville, KY 40280
888-560-8210
http://www.cbmw.com

Dad the Family Shepherd
P.O. Box 21445
Little Rock, AR 72221
800-234-3237
http://www.dtfs.org

Family Abuse Ministries
P.O. Box 6693
Bakersfield, CA 93306
661-319-0760
www.abuseministries.com

Family Life
P.O. Box 23840
Little Rock, AR 72221-3840
800-358-6329
http://www.familylife.com

Focus on the Family
Colorado Springs, CO 80995
800-232-6459
http://www.fotf.org

National Association for Christian Recovery
P.O. Box 215
Brea, CA 92822-0215
714-529-6227
http://www.christianrecovery.com/
http://www.nacronline.com/

National Coalition Against Domestic Violence
P.O. Box 18749
Denver, CO 80218
http://www.ncadv.org

National Domestic Violence Hotline
P.O. Box 161810
Austin, TX 78716
800-799-7233
http://www.ndvh.org

New Life Ministries
P.O. Box 650500
Dallas, TX 75265-0500
800-639-5433
http://www.newlife.com/

Promise Keepers
P.O. Box 103001
Denver, CO 80250-3001
303-964-7600
http://www.promisekeepers.org/

Shattered Men International
P.O. Box 166
Marion, IN 46952-0166
http://www.shatterdmen.com

Survivors of Spiritual Abuse
http://www.sosa.org/

U.S Department of Justice
Violence Against Women Office
810 7th Street, NW
Washington, DC 20531
202-307-6026
http://www.ojp.usdoj.gov/vawo/about.htm

Women of the Evangelical Lutheran Church of America
8765 W. Higgins Rd.
Chicago, IL 60631-4189
773-380-2730
http://www.elca.org/wo/

Women in Need
20 Mason Drive
Irvine, CA 92618
949-588-2946
http://www.womeninneed.org

Suggested Reading

Alsdurf, James and Alsdurf, Phyllis (1989). *Battered into Submission: The Tragedy of Wife Abuse in the Christian Home.* Downers Grove, IL: InterVarsity Press.

Cloud, Henry and Townsend, John (1999). *Boundaries in Marriage.* Grand Rapids, MI: Zondervan.

Dobson, James (1996). *Love Must Be Tough: Proven Hope for Families in Crisis.* Colorado Springs, CO: Word Books.

Fortune, Marie (1995). *Keeping the Faith: Guidance for Christian Women Facing Abuse.* San Francisco: Harper.

House, Wayne (Editor) (1990). *Divorce and Remarriage: Four Christian Views.* Downers Grove, IL: InterVarsity Press.

Jasinski, Jana and Williams, Linda (Editors) (1998). *Partner Violence: A Comprehensive Review of 20 Years of Research.* Thousand Oaks, CA: Sage.

Ketterman, Grace (1992). *Verbal Abuse: Healing the Hidden Wound.* Ann Arbor, MI: Servant Publications.

Kroeger, Catherine Clark and Beck, James (Editors) (1998). *Healing the Hurting: Giving Hope and Help to Abused Women.* Grand Rapids, MI: Baker House Books.

Miles, Al (2000). *Domestic Violence: What Every Pastor Needs to Know.* Minneapolis, MN: Fortress Press.

Missler, Nancy (1995). *Why Should I Be the First to Change?* Coeur d'Alene, ID: Koinonia House.

Peck, M. Scott (1997). *People of the Lie: The Hope for Healing Human Evil* (Second Edition). New York: Simon and Schuster.

Rinck, Margaret (1990). *Christian Men Who Hate Women.* Grand Rapids, MI: Zondervan.

Stonebraker, Bill (2000). *Spiritual Warfare in Marriage: Winning the Battle for a Good Marriage.* Honolulu, HI: Calvary Chapel.

Taves, Ann (Editor) (1989). *Religion and Domestic Violence in Early New England: The Memoirs of Abigail Abbot Bailey.* Bloomington, IN: Indiana University Press.

Weitzman, Susan (2000). *"Not to People Like Us": Hidden Abuse in Upscale Marriages.* New York: Basic Books.

Wheat, Ed and Perkins-Oakes, Gloria (1996). *Love Life for Every Married Couple.* Grand Rapids, MI: Zondervan.

Index

Order a copy of this book with this form or online at:
http://www.haworthpressinc.com/store/product.asp?sku=4568

FAMILY ABUSE AND THE BIBLE
The Scriptural Perspective

_____ in hardbound at $49.95 (ISBN:0-7890-1576-5)
_____ in softbound at $19.95 (ISBN: 0-7890-1577-3)

COST OF BOOKS_____

OUTSIDE USA/CANADA/
MEXICO: ADD 20%____

POSTAGE & HANDLING_____
*(US: $4.00 for first book & $1.50
for each additional book)
Outside US: $5.00 for first book
& $2.00 for each additional book)*

SUBTOTAL_____

in Canada: add 7% GST____

STATE TAX____
*(NY, OH & MIN residents, please
add appropriate local sales tax)*

FINAL TOTAL____
*(If paying in Canadian funds,
convert using the current
exchange rate, UNESCO
coupons welcome.)*

❏ **BILL ME LATER:** ($5 service charge will be added)
(Bill-me option is good on US/Canada/Mexico orders only;
not good to jobbers, wholesalers, or subscription agencies.)

❏ Check here if billing address is different from
shipping address and attach purchase order and
billing address information.

Signature_____

❏ **PAYMENT ENCLOSED: $**_____

❏ **PLEASE CHARGE TO MY CREDIT CARD.**

❏ Visa ❏ MasterCard ❏ Amex ❏ Discover
❏ Diner's Club ❏ Eurocard ❏ JCB

Account # _____

Exp. Date_____

Signature_____

Prices in US dollars and subject to change without notice.

NAME_____
INSTITUTION_____
ADDRESS_____
CITY_____
STATE/ZIP_____
COUNTRY_____ COUNTY (NY residents only)_____
TEL_____ FAX_____
E-MAIL_____

May we use your e-mail address for confirmations and other types of information? ❏ Yes ❏ No
We appreciate receiving your e-mail address and fax number. Haworth would like to e-mail or fax special
discount offers to you, as a preferred customer. **We will never share, rent, or exchange your e-mail address
or fax number.** We regard such actions as an invasion of your privacy.

Order From Your Local Bookstore or Directly From
The Haworth Press, Inc.
10 Alice Street, Binghamton, New York 13904-1580 • USA
TELEPHONE: 1-800-HAWORTH (1-800-429-6784) / Outside US/Canada: (607) 722-5857
FAX: 1-800-895-0582 / Outside US/Canada: (607) 722-6362
E-mail: getinfo@haworthpressinc.com
PLEASE PHOTOCOPY THIS FORM FOR YOUR PERSONAL USE.
www.HaworthPress.com

BOF02